Powerfully Pregnant

Donna Young N.D.
Traditional Midwife

Cover design by
Robert R Sewell, Jr.

First Printing July 2012

All Intellectual Property Rights belong exclusively to the author. No part of this publication may be copied, printed or reproduced in any manner without the written permission of Donna Young. Violations are punishable by both criminal and civil law.

Disclaimer: This book is intended for educational purposes only and is not intended to diagnose or prescribe for any disease or ailment. The information in this book is not intended to replace qualified health care professionals and does not promote unassisted child birth.

Dedication

To my father, for providing a lifetime
of direction in how to think

To my mother, for providing decades
of direction in what to study

Thanks, for believing in me.
I love and miss you both.

Appreciation

Thank you to my beautiful children who hold an honest appreciation for this lifestyle and the efforts going into it. You have missed many an activity or family gathering because Mom got called out on a birth and never once was there a moment of resentment by any of you, just the best wishes for every mother and child. Your devotion makes this work possible. Your unconditional support during the writing of this book has been noted and is very much appreciated. I love you all.

A special Thank You to Bear and Holt for picking up my workload at home over the last months, as I have been occupied with writing, and for being so excited and happy during the process. You are wonderful.

I am grateful to my clients for going the extra mile for a positive outcome. It takes heart and soul to do things right, day after day, for the wellbeing of yourself and your child. Without your efforts my knowledge is not worth having. I give knowledge; it is you who have put it into application. You do amazing! Also, the recipes shared within were donated by clients and loved ones who have put in many hours finding, making, or adjusting recipes to fit into diet and then shared them so generously. Thank you so much.

To Tabitha and Brooke for the hours of computer help and corrections that were needed. This book would never have been completed if it were not for your friendship, encouragement, donation of valuable time and precious input. Thank you so much.

Bob, Thank you for the cover design and the kind words along with and all the hours of various help throughout. Your friendship is priceless.

In special appreciation to those who donated their stories and photos for being so willing to help others. Thank you.

Never forgotten; for the intelligence, insight, humor, devotion and grit especially when I was consumed with finding solutions. I do.

About the Author
by Robert Sewell Jr.

Donna Young ND, is a Mother first and foremost, and a truly dedicated Traditional Midwife in a close second. Donna Young became a Certified Natural Health Counselor in 1988. She had completed her Naturopathic Doctor's degree in 1991. Donna Young has been delivering babies since 1995, with an impressive success rate.

Her exposure to the herbal world started under the wonderful example of her Mother and Father. It wasn't until her early adulthood that she had the opportunity to truly note the more desirable outcomes associated with natural approaches. These experiences drove her innermost passion to hone a program exclusively for natural home birthing. Many years of careful journal entries and photographs contributed to a clear view of her program. Donna Young is a highly respected Traditional Midwife and a very knowledgeable herbalist. Her dedication to structuring this program is above and beyond honorable.

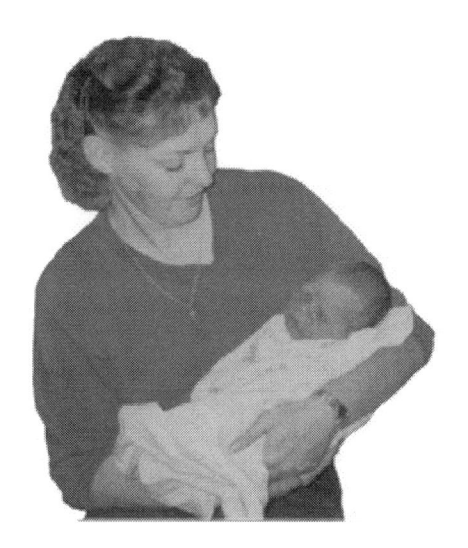

"Donna asks me sometimes how I am feeling and I reply *'Better than I did in my twenties. When my diet is Lily White there are no problems.'*"
Elizabeth ~ age 39

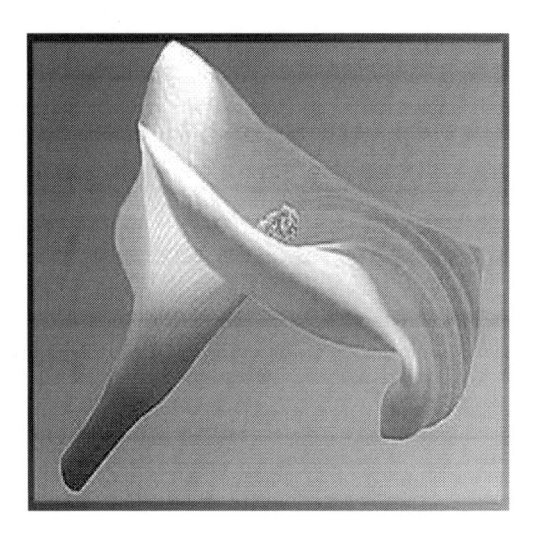

Lily White: Beyond reproach; blameless.

Foreword

Natural is defined as being within a state of nature. For several thousand years women have been giving birth in the natural setting of their living environment.

The living environment has an incredible influence within our lives. Having your baby at home is a symbolic gesture of love in the comfort of your surroundings. Choosing your environment for childbirth is a small fraction of what super charges the beginning of life. Every moment from conception to birth is an important contribution to the baby's health. In turn this directly attributes to the baby's incredible bond with parents after birth.

Powerfully Pregnant is a fine tuned and well practiced set of techniques that has proven time and time again, to have powerful and positive outcomes. Abiding by the process described within, you can be empowered to experience a more powerful pregnancy with incredible results after delivery. Starting a precious life is well deserving of such standards that exceed a lifetime, and for generations afterwards.

This book details natural pregnancy, and how nature intended it to be the most powerful experience in your lifetime. This is Powerfully Pregnant, and it is also the beginning of your beautiful journey.

Robert R. Sewell Jr.

TABLE OF CONTENTS

Title page	I
Intellectual Property Rights and Disclaimer	II
Dedication	III
Appreciation	IV
About the Author	V
Lily White	VI
Foreword by Robert Sewell, Jr.	VII
Table of Contents	VIII
1 Reason for Powerfully Pregnant	1

Pregnancy in History /Through the Eyes of my Father/Statistics/So What Happened? /The Journey that Lead to Powerfully Pregnant / Purpose of this Book/Short Stories

2 Explanation of Diet	11

Foods to be Avoided / Meal Time / Short story/Foods to Avoid-List /Foods to Eat Sparingly-List / Foods to Eat Freely-List /Short Stories

3 Supplements	22

Prenatal tea / Supplements Throughout Pregnancy /Beginning of Week 25/ Beginning of Week 35/ Beginning Week 39

4 Kala's Story	30
5 Exercises (with Megan)	39

Pelvic rocks / Squats / Butterflies/ Walking / Walking stairs /Kegels /Short Story

6 Heidi's Story	46
7 Prenatal Care	49

Urine test - Blood, Urobilinogen and Billirubin, Protein, Nitrites, Ketones, Glucose, Specific Gravity, pH, Leukocytes /Weight/Blood Pressure, Pulse/Check for edema/ Fundal measurement / Fetal Heart Tones and Cord Sounds/ Answer questions

8 Lyndsy's Story	58
9 Miscarriages	60

Emotional changes / Troubleshooting miscarriages, Estrogen, Lifting, Urinary Tract Infection, Low Blood Pressure - Anemia, Overheating, Thyroid, Environmental Toxins / After-Miscarriage Cleansing / Short Story

10 First Trimester	68

Breast Soreness/Constipation/Fatigue - Dizziness/Flatulence/Food Cravings/ Frequent Urination/ Headaches /Heartburn /Morning Sickness

11 Becky's Story	75
12 Second Trimester	78

Dry Skin/ Edema - Water Retention/Emotions/Gestational Diabetes /Hemorrhoids /High Blood Pressure / Infections / Restless Legs /Varicosities/Weight gain / Short Story

13 Edelweiss' Story	86
14 Third Trimester	92

Braxton Hicks Contractions/Braxton Hicks, Prior to Last Month/Braxton Hicks, Lack of /Breech Baby/False Labor/ Fear/Floating Baby/Insomnia/Muscle Cramps /Low Back Pain/ Premature Labor/Sciatica/ Slipped or Posterior Cervix /Stretch Marks/Short Stories

15 Tabitha's Story	101

16 Father's Section   104
    Understanding Her Emotions /She Complains a Lot/She is always Throwing Up / She has Weird Food Cravings / Her Breasts Hurt / She Doesn't Like Sex Anymore/ She Tosses and Turns all Night/She is Always Going to the Bathroom /Her Back Hurts/She seems so Sad / Will sex put Her into Labor? / Why the Internal Exams? / What is My Job During Labor and Delivery? / How Long do We Have to Wait to Have Sex After the Birth?

17 Mande's Story   113

18 Single Mother's Section   120

19 Melissa's Letter   124

20 Labor and Delivery   126
    Labor and Delivery Process, Start of Labor, Cervix, Effacement, Patterns, Spectators, Comfort, Pressure Points, Pushing, Crowning, Dilation of the Perineum, The Cord, Baby's First Breath, Delivery of the Placenta, Clean-up, Checking the Placenta / Reasons for Transport / Word of Advice /Patient Rights

21 Breast Issues   137
    To Relieve Pressure/Understanding the System/Resolve the Problem/Adjusting Butterfat Content of Breast Milk/Loss of Milk Supply/ Supplements

22 Elizabeth's Story   144

23 Erin's Story   146

24 Baby after the Birth   148
    APGAR /Documentation/Length/Head/Chest/ Vernix/Skin/The Head/Eyes/ First Cry/ Sucking Reflex/Breathing/Heart Rate/Digestion/ The Back/ Examining the Rectum/ Meconium/Checking the Hips/Checking Reflexes/ Treating the Cord/ Color/ Temperature/Holding Breath /Breast Feeding/ Umbilical Hernia/Rashes, Irritated Skin /Cradle Cap

25 Mother after the Birth   156
    Things to Watch / Supplements After the Birth / Beyond Supplements/ How Long to Wait to Have Sex After giving Birth

26 Pregnancy Journal   160
    My Powerfully Pregnant Journal/First Trimester/Second Trimester/Third Trimester/ The Birth / About Baby

27 Recipes   176
    The Program/Changing Recipes to Fit/Breakfast Ideas/Lunch and Dinner Ideas/ Salads/Dressings, Spreads, Misc. /Desserts and Treats/ Know your ingredients / Short Stories

~1~
REASON FOR POWERFULLY PREGNANT

Pregnancy in History

I once read a midwifery book, written by A.I. Coffin, MD in 1853, called *Treatise on Midwifery and the Diseases of Women and Children*, 7th edition (which was used as a training tool at BYU). In this book Dr. Coffin tells of the problems and successes of pregnancy and childbirth. I would like to reflect on some of the things I found interesting in his book.

In the preface he says, *"The duty appears to have devolved upon us to tear those impediments from the minds of our fair readers, and if possible to induce every mother to properly instruct and direct her daughter in all things that is requisite for her to know. Were she thus properly informed, there would be but little use for that class of men called doctors. And why should she not know? Why not understand herself, and everything pertaining to herself? Also in rearing of children, in which, by accordance with the laws of nature, and pursuing her unvarying dictates, little difficulty is experienced in relieving their wants and removing their maladies. But when art is substituted for nature, where everything is recommended that comes in direct contact with their natural wants, and the healthy action of their systems; and when at the same time the mothers are taught to believe all this to be right, it is not to be wondered at that so many die in infancy, from the numerous maladies to which it is said they are subject; yet most of those afflictions have been brought on by want of the proper knowledge of feeding, clothing and nursing the child."* He goes on to say, *"In the practice of midwifery, in every part of God's fair earth, except where it is said science and civilization prevail, is directed by the laws, and under the sole superintendence, of Nature. In those districts there seldom or ever occurs a death, either with the mother or child; and in many places there is not any attendant, either as nurse of midwife; and what is still better, the mother suffers little or no pain."*

Dr. Coffin states, that in Paris, over a period of time there were 70,000 women who delivered at a 'lying-in' hospital, which is where women would go to deliver their baby. Tradition had it that men, including doctors, should not see the private parts or uncovered body of another man's wife so the women would be given a room with a bed and wash basin and deliver her own baby. If problems occurred, beyond the capabilities of the mother, then the woman would go to the door and request help otherwise she was left alone to deliver her own child. Of the 70,000 women that delivered at a 'lying-in' hospital, only 12 women requested help. Personally, I thought it was wonderful that the other 69,988 women were able to successfully deliver without any assistance.

Dr. Coffin says, *"--that the further society is removed from the influence of the medical profession, the less disease they suffer; and the more they follow the laws and dictates of Nature, the less their sufferings during pregnancy"*.

Dr. Coffin discusses the management of pregnancy, which included five things;

"First--The strictest temperance and regularity in diet, sleeping, exercise and amusements are necessary to be observed by those who have reasons to dread abortions.

Second--Overheating, irregular passions and costiveness, should be constantly guarded against.

Third--The hazards of shocks, from falls in walking, or riding, from bruises in crowds, or frights from bustle, should be avoided with the utmost circumspection.

Fourth--The dress ought to be loose and easy; tight lacing is injurious at every period of pregnancy."

"Fifth--Pregnant women require free, pure air; their inclinations should be gratified by every reasonable indulgence; and their spirits kept up by cheerful company, and a variety of objects, that their minds may always be composed and happy."

Dr. Coffin makes an interesting comment, *"Our readers will remark that throughout the whole of the above details, which are strictly in accordance with the doctrines of the schools, the only midwife is NATURE, or the natural powers exerted by the system, without the least assistance from any other source; and further, in our opinion, there is not one case in a thousand but what would do better left to its own natural powers, than if interfered with in the ordinary manner of schools."*

"Young women, apparently well proportioned, of a lax fibre, and healthy constitution, may be presumed to have easy, favorable labours."

Dr. Coffin describes assisting the birth itself and he says, "At *this period, the patient should be held under no restraint, but permitted to walk or rest, until the pains become more severe; when she should be placed upon the bed on her left side, with her knees drawn up, and we have found it useful, as the labour advances, to separate them with a pillow; something for the feet to rest against, will also afford great assistance. Having thus placed the patient in as comfortable a situation as circumstances allow, and guarded against everything that may disturb or annoy, we must wait with patience until the natural pains have brought the head of the child to the external orifice, when assistance is generally required to support the perineum (the soft part between the two passages). Which is done by slight pressure on that part with the palm of the hand. When the head is born, we must take care that its position, in relation to the mother, shall be such as to not injure it. This is natural labour; and in most every instance women require no more assistance than we have above described, in fact, as we have before said, and we feel that we cannot too strongly impress it on the minds of our readers, that mechanical assistance in nine hundred and ninety-nine cases out of a thousand, does more harm than good. That we can assist by assisting nature is certain; but then this can be done without wrapping everything in mystery, and rendering obscure that which it is most to the interest of the patient to know; for bear in mind, it is the patient that has to perform the work, not the doctor."*

Dr. Coffin has a most interesting thought when he pleads with the women of England by saying, *"Women of England! will you longer submit to such a system of fraud and deception? Will you still suffer all your finer feelings to be outraged by the admission of a man into the most secret recesses of your chamber, under the pretence of being absolutely necessary to your recovery? Will you so far sacrifice your self-respect, your innate modesty and sense of delicacy, at the shrine of custom or fashion, to uphold a monstrous monopoly? Can you be so willfully blind to your own comforts, so ignorant of the great fact that nature is the best midwife, and can and will accomplish all that is necessary, as to countenance on of that class who tells you 'Oh, I did something for you before I went away which made it quite unnecessary for any further assistance'. No! we feel confident you will no longer submit to this degrading practice! You will arise in your beauty, your power, and your might, and loudly and fervently protest against it; you will break the fetters if an unnatural custom, pluck the scales from off your eyes, and see, think, and judge for yourselves, and in so doing act with such determination as shall at once and for ever sweep this 'secret history of adultery' this immodest deformity, from the surface of this fair land."*

"There are more than sixty forms of disease to which it is said children are subject during their young existence; yet we can assure our readers that, by due observance of the mother, before birth, in keeping up a healthy action of her own system, in nineteen cases out of twenty none of those forms of disease will exist in her offspring".
Throughout Dr. Coffin's book, he stood firm in his beliefs that nature was the best midwife and

with the right guidelines a woman could give birth with little or no pain and with very few complications and that was over 150 years ago.

Through the Eyes of my Father
After I had been delivering babies for over a decade my father and I had a discussion about childbirth. He was confused as to why women needed a birth attendant because it was such a natural and simple process that anyone should be able to handle it alone. I explained there were risks and problems that women could not handle alone, and it was far safer to have a knowledgeable birth attendant present. My father, who was about 75 years old at the time, told me a story that left a lasting impression on him.

When my father was 18 years old (1944) he was working as a cowboy for a ranch in Southern Utah. The ranch bordered an Indian reservation with the Colorado River being the boundary on that side with the ranch house about 35 miles in from the river. The owner of the ranch asked my father to go with him to find out who was taking some of his cattle. They rode about five miles and came upon the remains of a cow that had been butchered. Both being excellent trackers, they followed the tracks for another ten miles and found a place where a woman had given birth. My father and the rancher continued on, until they caught up with the group of people just as they were nearing the river. My father and the rancher questioned the men in the group about the beef and came to an agreement that their people were certainly in need of the food, but in the future they would come to the ranch and allow the rancher to choose the beef they took instead of taking the more expensive breeding stock. As the conversation was nearing an end, the rancher told the men that he knew there was a baby with them, and he wanted to see the baby to insure its safety. After some persuasion, a young Indian girl stepped out from behind the wagon with the baby in her arms. The baby was healthy and content. They confirmed that the young mother had walked into where the cattle were, to help with the kill and preparation of the meat the night before. The baby was born during the night and the following day she had started the trek back with the rest of her group. They were just a few miles from their camp and she was comfortable with crossing the river and going the rest of the way home. She had no signs of excess bleeding, weakness, or fatigue, and her color was good. She assured my father and the rancher she was in good health and wanted to continue her trip home. My father concluded from this experience, that it should be as easy for any woman to give birth, as it was for his range stock who very rarely suffered any form of complications.

A few days after telling the story, my father watched a video of two births I had recently attended. He watched intently as these babies were delivered without undo stress, and both of the mothers were in peaceful control during labor. Both babies were delivered completely clean with no blood from tears, and took breath spontaneously. When the video was over he thought for a few minutes and then said, "That is exactly how every baby should come into this world." From that moment on, my father became one of my greatest supporters.

Statistics
According to the latest US National Vital Statistics Report (2006)

> *Number of vaginal deliveries: 2,929,590*
> *Number of Cesarean deliveries: 1,321,054*
> *Percent of all deliveries by Cesarean: 31%*
> *Infant Mortality rate: 6.69 deaths per 1,000 live births*
> *In 2006, diabetes during pregnancy (diabetes diagnosed both prior to and during pregnancy), was reported at a rate of 42.3 per 1,000 women, (just over 4 percent) compared with 38.5 per 1,000 in 2005*

"The low birthweight (LBW) rate rose from 8.2 to 8.3 percent for 2005–2006, the sixth consecutive year of increase and the highest level reported in the U.S. in four decades."
Pregnancy-associated hypertension is the more common of the two conditions occurring in 2006 at a rate of 39.1 per 1,000, compared with 10.8 for chronic hypertension
These data show that in 2006, 13 percent of all mothers gained less than 16 pounds, which is considered inadequate for most women, and 21 percent had weight gains of more than 40 pounds, considered excessive for all women. Thus, approximately one-third of all mothers had weight gains outside of the guidelines, regardless of their height.

Prenatal care utilization had improved for all groups between 1990 and 2003, especially among those whom historically had less timely care. These gains were linked to the expansion of Medicaid for pregnant women in the late 1980s; studies suggest that more recent changes to welfare and Medicaid policy might limit further improvements in timely care.

For 2006, the rate of induction of labor rose one percent, from 222.7 to 225.3 per one thousand births in 2005 (or 22.3 and 22.5 percent of all births). It has been suggested that the shifting of deliveries towards earlier gestational ages may be due to increased use of induction, and other obstetric interventions such as cesarean delivery.

The total cesarean delivery rate for 2006, 31.1 percent, is the highest level ever reported in the United States. This is a three percent increase from the 2005 rate (30.3 percent). The continuing rise in the total cesarean rate is a result of trends in the primary cesarean rate and the rate of VBAC.

In 2006, a National Institutes of Health expert panel recommended, that non-medically indicated cesareans should not be performed for pregnancies of less than 39 weeks of gestation or, for women desiring several children.

"The preterm birth rate rose again in 2006 to 12.8 percent of all births."

The low birth weight (LBW) rate also continued to rise, climbing to eight point three percent in 2006, this was the highest level in four decades.

According to Wikipedia:
The mean stillbirth rate in the United States is approximately 1 in 115 births, which is roughly 26,000 stillbirths each year, or on an average one every 20 minutes. Prospective studies, using very sensitive early pregnancy tests, have found that 25% of pregnancies are miscarried by the sixth week from the woman's last menstrual period (LMP). Clinical miscarriages, those occurring after the sixth week LMP, occur in 8% of all U.S. pregnancies.

Infant mortality is 630 per 100,000 live births or 6. 3 per 1000 live births.

So What Happened?
There have been a lot of changes. Many are quick to blame the change on the medical, and legal professional's for the added complications, the invasive procedures, the laws that mandate to protect the medical industry, and the chemical medications. In my opinion, that is not what forced the high complication rate of pregnancy and birthing in the U.S. I believe that it was women who changed. It was women who changed their lifestyle. It was women who got office jobs, became sedentary, and started hiring the physical things in their world out, instead of doing for themselves. Women started mopping their floors standing up and not spending time on their hands and knees. Women changed their diet from wholesome foods to fast foods. They started

eating for speed and flavor instead of nutrition. Women became addicted to junk food and other things that are more obviously harmful to their bodies such as drugs, alcohol, and tobacco. The medical professional's simply changed to accommodate the needs we developed as we changed. And the laws changed to fit the current situation.

In order to change the outcome women must change themselves. A doctor/midwife cannot find a reason to transport, or the need to perform a cesarean if our bodies are performing the way nature intended them to work. Women must step up to the plate and assume responsibility for their actions, their pregnancies, their bodies, and their outcome. Only then can we change the statistics to an acceptable level in our great nation.

How do we change ourselves, when we don't know what we are doing wrong? We must become educated. Once we become educated about our health, we have direction. Once we have direction, the personal responsibility becomes much easier and the ability to succeed is then within our reach.

The Journey that Lead to This Program
I was about 17 years old when my mother had her seventh major surgery in three years. According to Mother, she was laying in a hospital after her surgery and a friend of hers, Judy, came in and dropped an herb book in her lap and said, "While you have time here, why don't you figure out what you can do for yourself instead of letting the doctors whittle you to death". Judy then turned and walked out. My mother picked up the book and began reading. This was a major turning point in Mother's life and though none of us realized it, that moment would eventually change our entire family, for generations.

For the first few years I somewhat heckled my mother over her new found knowledge. She tried to teach me and I would say things like, "What do you do? Do you put the herbs on a tree stump under a full moon, do your heebie-jeebies and they magically make you better?" She would patiently say, "Someday you will understand".

In 1976, at 21 years of age, I was pregnant with my first child. My husband had full medical coverage, and only 'the best' would do for our baby. I traveled 100 miles to a specialist that had a lot of letters behind his name. He had just started his own practice and was very personable and willing to take time to answer questions. He strongly suggested that I consume a diet of milk, beef, and potatoes and that I exercise regularly. I followed his instructions to the letter, after all, I had been raised on a beef and potatoes diet and so it fell right into place. During this pregnancy; I had four months of morning sickness, a respiratory infection (that lasted months), and then wrapped it up with a 14 hour labor and delivery, an episiotomy and an, "Atta girl!!" from the doctor for doing such a great job. It took me weeks to heal up, but I lost the extra weight within a few weeks, and the doctor told me I was doing great, because pregnancy is such a traumatic ordeal for our bodies. I was happy because, we had a beautiful little girl to show for it and she was well worth the price I paid.

In 1978, I was pregnant with the second child and went back to the same specialist. He told me I should consume a diet of milk and seafood three times a day and I asked, "What? What happened to meat and potatoes? Why the change?" He answered, "New research." This seemed odd to me, after all the years of pregnancy, since Adam and Eve, why would the rules change now? I decided, "Well, I like seafood so what the heck". I went home and told my husband what the good doctor said and my husband did his part to see that my needs were met. Through this pregnancy I had; five solid months of morning sickness, yeast infections, respiratory infections, and fatigue. Near the end of the pregnancy I went into the doctor and told him, "I have not felt the baby move in almost two weeks". He did an ultrasound and said, "Oh, it is just a lazy boy. Don't worry, everything is okay". A few days later, I went into labor and had a 16 hour labor that felt totally different than the first. We had to do an emergency transport to the local hospital where this baby was born with another episiotomy. I asked my doctor, "Why the difference?" and he told me, "There is no method to the madness. There is no pattern to hard pregnancies or deliveries. Sometimes they are easier and sometimes they are harder and you never know what you are going to get until it is over." This confused me, my father had taught me that when cows are pregnant they need to have a different diet. "Don't over feed them or they have trouble calving." "Keep their diet as natural as possible." He pointed out the ease which wildlife delivered their babies, if there was no outside interference. If there is a pattern to cows, horses, dogs, cats, deer, and elk there had to be a pattern with people. We had to be doing something to cause it.

At six weeks old, my second baby was still sleeping 20 hours a day, and the pediatrician was telling me that it was normal for some babies to sleep that much. Again I am told, "he is just a lazy boy and will probably grow out of it". He was a beautiful child and I was grateful to have him, but I was confused about whether my change in diet had something to do with his fatigue. I was haunted by the attitude that the diet had nothing to do with the outcome.

In the spring 1981, my first-born came down with asthma, at four years of age. She was in and out of the hospital on a regular basis for the next few years. She was taken to specialist after specialist and was on over 30 different medications on a regular basis. She was frail and weak and finally one day in 1986, as she lay in the hospital, the doctor took me out in the hall to have a very frank discussion with me. "Donna," he said "She has run a long, hard battle but she has lost and the only thing keeping her alive is the fact that you refuse to let go. If you would just go in there and give her permission she could slip into God's hands and her suffering would be over." I looked at him and said I needed a few minutes. I walked down the hall and called my mother, who was living in Idaho. I asked, "Mom, realistically, is there anything that can be done? Is there anything that can save her life?" My mom responded, "Yes, if you are willing to change your attitude." I broke to tears and said, "Do tell me what the hell my attitude has to do with her asthma!" She very calmly said, "You have to stop handing someone else an insurance card, and asking them to assume responsibility for the child God placed in your arms." It took me a matter of seconds to realize that she was right. I had been guilty of exactly what she said.

I walked back down the hall where the doctor met me, and asked him if he wanted to go with me to talk to my little girl. He said, "Yes." He was a quiet man that had grown very fond of her over the previous four years and it showed in his face that he also, was feeling the pain of her illness. He stood at the end of the bed as I walked around to the other side, and spoke to her, "Sweetheart, are you awake?" "Yes" she replied. "Then open your eyes and look at me." I told her in a more firm tone. She opened her eyes and looked up at me. "Sweetheart, if you die I will kick your butt! We are going to take you to go see Grandma" I told her. Then I turned to the doctor and said, "If she's going to be taken, it is not going to be from a place like this. Check her out of here." The doctor, who had always been very kind and caring yielded to my wishes and checked her out of the hospital. Within 48 hours I had her in Idaho where I was living near my parents and they willingly helped in every way they could.

They gave me books to read about prescription medications so that I could read about what each one was doing to her body, both good and bad. My parents had shelf after shelf of herbal and natural health books and I read everything they had on asthma. I decided I would change her diet, use supplements, and have a complete change in attitude about my children's health and my role in it. I still stop and think now and then about how grateful I am for the day Judy changed the direction of our family's health. She saved many lives that day and was the first to lay foundation for the thoughts of homebirth. I am grateful that my parents had heeded to her advice and changed their own lives and started me on the road to a life of self-sufficiency in health. I started my formal studies for a Naturopathic degree, primarily to be able to help my own family. At the time, I was a medical receptionist and this gave me the opportunity to see both sides of this controversial subject of medical vs. natural. Best of all, my little girl would live to grow up and become a healthy adult.

In 1987, I was pregnant with child number three. I went to my father and asked him, "Which do you think is best for childbirth? Hospital or home births?" His response was simple, "Which cows have fewer calving problems? Range cows or dairy cows?" I answered, "Range cows, they never seem to have problems, and even old dairy cows tend to have complications." "That is right." He said, "But why?" I answered, "Because they have less interference." Dad said, "That is right, go to where you have the least interference to have your child." I was very at peace with that response. I decided to call a Naturopath who lived in Idaho Falls. I had met with this Naturopath briefly at about 18 years of age and liked him so I asked him if he would deliver my baby. He agreed but gave no dietary advice and he gave no supplement advice. I began studying to figure out what I needed to do to have a healthier pregnancy than the two before. The end result was one month of morning sickness, minimal weight gain and a four-hour labor and delivery. I knew I was on the right track but needed more. This son was beautiful, healthy and developed physically, mentally and emotionally at a very pleasing pace. By this time I was working as a Certified Natural Health Counselor in a shop with my parents and health was a primary focus for all of us.

In 1990, I became pregnant with child number four. I had very little morning sickness and again I had a four-hour labor. For my fifth pregnancy, I called a midwife that lived closer. And as I worked with her, she saw me regularly and I followed her advice. She used supplements, but her dietary instructions were, "It does not matter what you eat, just eat! Big babies are healthy babies!" Sure enough, I had lots of weight gain with a shorter delivery and a much bigger baby. "Hmmm..." I thought. This showed to have its pros and cons as there was a ton of weight to get rid of, but it was a 30 minute delivery and I was back to work after the weekend, four days after the birth.

I was finding common denominators with each pregnancy and the health of each child. My father had pressed an issue all my life, "If you have a problem more than once look for common denominators." I watched clients and kept notes on which diets and supplements brought what outcomes. I began watching women who had common problems and then began to see what else they had in common. I was forever watching for clues to the 'mystery of pregnancy'.

In 1999, I was pregnant with little number six. By this time I had been a Naturopath in Idaho for eight years and had been delivering babies for almost five years. I had worked out all the kinks in diet and supplements. I had no morning sickness, no excess weight gain and at 44 years of age, I felt better during this pregnancy than I did in my twenties to show for it. I decided by the fifth month that I wanted to deliver my own baby and was preparing to have enough strength to follow through with the task. I asked someone to be with me when I delivered, for safety reasons and on the night I went into labor, my witness laid on the couch asleep and I was talking on the phone when my back started hurting. A heating pad relieved the pressure, but I decided to go take a hot bath to relax my back. I ran the bath and as soon as I got in, there was a strong contraction, but only lasted 30 seconds. I called my witness to come in, and as she walked through the door she asked if there was anything she could do. I asked her to time the contraction that was just starting. It lasted two minutes and 40 seconds (a very long contraction as they usually do not last over 90 seconds). She commented how nicely I had handled the contractions and just then my third contraction started. I leaned my head back, and thought about how, 'if these continue to get harder I will need to get out of the tub'. Just then my body went into a bearing down push and her little head was born. I felt her trying to take her first breath, while her body was still inside me, so I pushed her out into my hands and brought her up out of the water. I tipped her upside down to assist the water out of her mouth and nose as she turned her little head and looked straight at me. In that instant I fell in love with her. Then I turned her upright and put her to my heart and held her close. A cherished moment for sure! After a few minutes of cuddle time, the witness took my baby, still connected to me with the cord and we got out of the tub. We walked around the corner and sat down on the edge of the bed. It had been 10 minutes since I had hung up the phone. In my eyes this was the perfect birth. I was back into my pre-pregnancy jeans in three days without any signs of postpartum depression. All in all, I knew we had certainly found the perfect program to have a baby.

I continue to watch clients and see the parallels between diet and their outcomes. I'm always searching for supplements and foods that are the most beneficial for mothers and babies. The program is customized to each situation as each mother has her own history and needs. There are basics that never change and then there are things that need to be fine-tuned.

Purpose of this Book
I am always disappointed when I hear of someone who has been told by her healthcare provider that all of her ailments, discomforts and problems are a normal part of pregnancy and she 'should just accept it' or 'there is nothing that can be done about it'. There is usually something that can be done. Humans are the only beings on the face of this earth that accept disease as a natural course. Why would we accept illness and disease as normality? Why would we accept a 30%+ c-section rate and even higher miscarriage and complication rates as normal? We should be reading and studying to figure out what we can do for ourselves. There are always solutions, no matter what the problem, there has to be a solution. This book contains many of the solutions that I give to my own clientele, hoping to give women motivation to search deeper for solutions instead of accepting problems as inevitable.

The purpose of this book is to help you with enough knowledge to help yourself through a healthier pregnancy. No one can do it for you, it is total personal responsibility. If you are eating right and exercising, even the toughest health issues can be improved upon.

If you have a (personal or family) history of weight gain, infections, high blood pressure, immune deficiency, or any other heath problems you can improve your well-being. You even have the power to change the health of your children by eating with a conscious focus on nutrition. Once your child is born you can do them a great favor by teaching them to eat healthy so that the next generation can follow through, and become healthier than the last.

Children learn what their parents teach them and as parents, we have the responsibility to teach our children how to be healthy and to lay a foundation for a better future. I believe we can change the world one meal at a time. If we learn to avoid processed, and unfriendly foods, our bodies will be healthier and work more efficiently. Personal responsibility is the cornerstone to all health, whether it is during pregnancy, or at any other time in our lives. I have provided knowledge, but it is up to each individual to follow through with that knowledge and put it into action. Going the extra mile to be healthy is worth more than most can imagine and it takes a change of attitude and commitment.

This program can help to educate you about what is happening to your body during pregnancy. It will allow you to understand what foods are going to work for you, and which ones are going to work against you. If you are willing to follow the instructions in this book then it can teach you how to manage your pregnancy so you can generally prevent things like breech birth, or prolonged labors. No matter the nationality, the race, the religion, or the economic situation, this program empowers women to take control of their own health.

You can feel empowered with the birth of your child, because you will have more knowledge, strength, and control enabling you to make logical decisions.

My expectation for this program is, for every woman who follows it to the letter, to have;

1. The most perfect and wonderful pregnancy and delivery possible for her.
2. Improve upon her previous pregnancies and births.
3. Have more control of the outcome.
4. Empower each woman with enough knowledge and strength that she will embrace her birth experience.
5. Have solutions to problems.
6. Have knowledge to go through her pregnancy and birth the way she intends.

~~~~~A Short Story~~~~~

One day, a 17-year old girl came into my office and asked me to deliver her baby. I objected, because history had taught me that teenagers do not usually follow instructions. She promised that she would do whatever it took to have me deliver her baby. We talked and finally she broke into tears, "You don't understand, my entire family has very long and difficult labors. They all labor for 24 to 48 hours. I cannot go through that, I can't go through a 24-hour labor." "Please don't turn me away." I looked at the sincerity in her eyes and finally said, "I will take you on, but the first time you fail to follow instructions or the first time I see a problem you have to go to the hospital. Do you understand me?" "Yes, yes! I promise," she squealed. She was a beautiful girl who had wonderful family support as well as the support of her husband. I was a little concerned because she was not yet developed and very petite. She would need to mature during this pregnancy, but if she followed instructions I knew she would be okay. She was attentive to diet and kept all of her prenatal appointments. She did everything I asked of her and I began to see her mature physically and mentally. I knew that her and her husband would accommodate the needs of their child. Finally the day of her baby's birth arrived, she labored with grace and a cheerful attitude. Her husband whispered words of encouragement to her during labor and after a four-hour labor she gave birth to a beautiful daughter, cutting the time of her other family member's delivery times down to one-sixth. As young as this couple was, they are a perfect example for couples of all ages.

~~~~~A Short Story~~~~~

After having five children, I realized that I knew little more about childbirth than I did after having my first. I had one medical doctor, one naturopath and three midwives, each working on one or more of my five pregnancies. None of them felt a need to explain to me the changes that were taking place in my body during pregnancy or delivery. I read quite a few books on the subject of pregnancy, but was still misinformed and confused. Don't get me wrong, these were all super-nice people and did their jobs, but they just did not see the importance in sharing knowledge. Sometimes I felt their lack of sharing information, equated to a lack of knowledge and sometimes attendants crossed boundaries that should never have been crossed.

After having one of my babies I lay in bed, all alone in the room, for over an hour without anyone with me. I was not offered anything to eat or drink, not taken to the bathroom, not asked if I was bleeding or having problems. Nothing. Finally, the attendant walked by the bedroom door and I said, "Excuse me, where is my baby?" "Oh", he replied "The midwife is breastfeeding him." "What?!! Are you kidding me? I want my baby!" I was horribly offended that she would take it upon herself to breastfeed my new son that I had not even been given opportunity to hold yet. I was told that she thought she was doing me a favor because I was probably tired after that four hour labor. A birth attendant never has the right to make those kinds of decisions. The mother always has boundaries and they need to be respected.

When I started delivering babies, I felt very strongly that each woman should be taught what was going on in her body and what she could do to assist in the process for a better outcome and a mother's boundaries should always be respected. Sometimes, my personal experiences that formed my opinion of what was important, were based on positive experiences. Other times they were based on experiences that instilled protectiveness to make sure other women did not go through the same kinds of experiences I had.

Close to my due date with one of my babies, the midwife had a feeling that I needed to be checked. She arrived around eleven in the evening and cheerfully asked to do an exam. I thought to myself, "Oh my gosh! It is late and I have been up since early morning, I am tired and ready to go to bed." She talked for a little bit and then put the blood pressure cuff on my arm and started to take my blood pressure. She no sooner got it pumped up when I had a contraction that doubled me over. "Oh, how did she do that?!" I wondered. I had several more contractions, 90 seconds apart, and she started using pressure points to ease the pain. She then went to the phone to call the other midwife and as she was walking back across the floor my water broke. She ran down the hall and told the assistant, "Get the sheets on this bed we are having a baby now!" She came back down the hall and escorted me to the bedroom at the end of the hall. I reached for the bathroom door and told her I needed to go into the bathroom. She told me, "No". "Oh, you don't understand, I really need to go" I begged. She refused and told me to go into the bedroom. I sat down on the edge of the bed and went directly into a bearing down push. She got in my face and started blowing in my face and my contraction stopped. She took the next 60-90 seconds to get me in a position to deliver my baby. My baby boy was born on the next contraction. If it had not been for her intuitiveness, I would have probably had that baby on the toilet, alone. I was grateful for her being in tune with me, and having the strength to tell me 'no' when I started to make a wrong decision.

The midwives were gone within an hour after he was born, never to be heard from again. I felt it would have been nice to get a phone call showing some kind of interest in my condition and in our new baby, in case there was a problem, but that did not happen. The child-bearing experiences are some of the most important times of a woman's life and they need to be positive experiences.

NOTES_____
_____
_____
_____
_____
_____
_____
_____
_____
_____

~2~
EXPLANATION OF DIET

One of the greatest misconceptions in our modern world is that a healthy pregnancy is measured by the amount of weight gained. Weight should not be used as a way to measure health, rather by the quality of nutrients we are putting into our body and the end results. When we choose to eat nutrient dense foods our body begins to thrive, is more energetic, stronger, and leaner. A woman should never have to worry about counting calories, fat, or carbohydrates. When choosing to eat a healthy diet, a woman's body, whether she is over-weight, at a healthy weight, or under-weight will be able to regulate to a healthy weight. During pregnancy, a woman should never go hungry and should always eat when she feels like eating. Eating two to four meals per day with snacks in between.

Through years of experience I have found that the body works very efficiently when given the proper nutrition to work with. I have also found that foods that are lacking in nutrition have an adverse affect on the body. Every part of the body has its own nutritional needs just as every wholesome food has its own nutritional profile. When a wholesome food is eaten the body has the proper nutrition, which results in improved health.

Herbs and Supplements are a concentrated food for the purpose of nutritional support into a specific area of the body. Herbs are like vitamins and other supplements, they are to supplement the diet, but not replace diet. Many of the herbs can be used as culinary spices such as garlic, onion, fennel etc. Taking herbs in food form is as good, if not better than taking them in supplement form.

The dietary guidelines I suggest for most, especially during pregnancy, are as follows with the reasons indicated.

Foods to be Avoided

NO SUGAR brown sugar, white sugar, powdered sugar, raw sugar, and no processed sugar of any kind or anything ending in "ose" as an added or primary ingredient (fructose, lactose, glucose etc.). This does not include foods that have naturally occurring sugars in them such as fruits.

NO SYNTHETIC SWEETENERS like aspartame and sucralose. Synthetic sweeteners are all man-made sweeteners and are considered a foreign substance to the body. There have been syndromes associated with most artificial sweeteners.

Sugar lowers the immune system making it hard for the body to fight off disease and illness. "Every bite matters", an example is, if a person comes down with a cold and is following dietary guidelines the symptoms are alleviated in a couple of days. If they decide to ingest sugar the symptoms usually return within a short time and if inflicted with the cold the second time it has been found more difficult to alleviate the symptoms. People who eat sugar on a regular basis have even more difficulty alleviating symptoms.

Gestational diabetes, diabetes, and hypoglycemia are all too common in today's lifestyle due to the abundant sugar intake. Women who eat sugar during pregnancy are more prone to have babies with larger bone structure (this is usually more common after their first baby). Bigger bone structure makes pushing more difficult, increases the length of time baby is in the birth canal, and increases the chances of a tear.

I have found that women who consume sugar during their pregnancies are more prone to hemorrhage. The increased hemorrhaging is partially due to tearing but is also caused from the blood lacking integrity (the blood does not clot as well) if sugar is eaten.

Sugar turns acidic in the body increasing heartburn and acid reflux. Sugar also lowers pain tolerance, causing greater suffering during labor and delivery. A primary reason for high pain tolerance during child birth is the absence of sugar.

Acceptable Replacements
Honey
Stevia
Pure maple syrup
Molasses
Any natural sweetener

Caution: Honey, pure maple syrup and other concentrated sugars may not be acceptable for anyone who has gestational diabetes.

If the blood sugar has a tendency to drop and you have cravings try balancing it by eating more protein and fruits instead of foods containing sugar.

In all the women who have followed this diet, I have never had a single case of gestational diabetes, pre-eclampsia, high blood pressure, excess weight gain, depression or low pain tolerance. The women following these dietary guidelines have babies with an average birth weight of seven pounds (first time mothers and petite women's babies tend to be a little smaller); they rarely get stretch marks, little if any morning sickness, and no yeast infections. These women are strong, healthy and energetic as a rule!

NO CARBONATION soda, sparkling mineral water, sparkling fruit juice, etc., (nothing with a bubble should go into the body).

Carbonation has a tendency to shut down the liver and kidneys. The kidneys, liver, and spleen make up the filtering system in the body and if compromised can cause any disorder associated with them to be more prevalent. This becomes an issue with high blood pressure, water retention, toxemia, allergies, and infections.

Acceptable replacements
Clean water
Herbal Tea
Low-Acid Fruit Juice (100% juice, with no added sugar)
Water and Herbal teas should make up at least 75% of the fluid intake.

NO DAIRY including any milk that is produced from any animal. Commercially produced dairy products are loaded with hormones, antibiotics, mucous and infection. Extra hormones during pregnancy, especially bovine estrogen, can cause contractions and should be avoided. Progesterone is the relaxing hormone produced by the body to hold the pregnancy by not allowing the uterus to contract. Second hand antibiotics, found in dairy, compromises the immune system. Hormones are given to female cows to increase production of milk, making the cow produce more than nature would allow. A large amount of hormones come out in the cow's milk and are ingested by the consumer.

Organic milk does not contain antibiotics or added hormones, but still contains high amounts of mucous and infection. Milk is mucous forming which causes morning sickness and headaches. The immune system is already compromised during pregnancy, because the body is taking care of you and a new life. Putting more infection into the body will further compromise the immune system and overload the filtering system (kidneys, liver, and spleen).

Milk products that are combined with a sweetener(s) are even harder on the body. Things like ice cream and yogurt most frequently are the cause of morning sickness, sinus infections, digestive issues, and respiratory issues.

As a midwife, I remove most dairy products from a woman's diet, from conception to birth, and leave it optional after delivery. The exception to dairy is block, naturally aged, cheeses because they are the least damaging and are also a good source of protein. Unless a woman is having a hard time with morning sickness, constipation, digestive issues, respiratory problems, or headaches the naturally aged, block cheeses are fine.

Acceptable Replacements
Rice Milk
Coconut Milk
Almond Milk

NO GROUND GRAINS (FLOUR) this includes breads, pasta, cookies, tortillas, and even whole grain flour. If there is any kind of grain flour (rice, wheat, barley, rye, oat, etc.) in the ingredients then it is off limits. Yes, this includes homemade breads and sprouted grain breads because we have found them to have the same effects on pregnancy and labor as any other breads made with flour.

Grains are supposed to do their work inside the digestive tract, in a whole, cracked, or rolled state. In the form of a true whole grain, grains can be eaten as often as desired without any negative effects. Nowhere in nature do we find flour. We find grains whole and they get broken down with the teeth while being chewed. The whole grains provide fiber and nutrients that are to be taken in gradually as they travel through the digestive tract. Once the grain has been ground to a powder (flour) state, it crosses the intestinal/blood barrier and stores as fat presenting itself, primarily, as a shelf of excess weight across the hips, thighs and torso.

Flours are one of the largest factors for an excessive weight gain for most ladies and puts the big, chubby cheeks and extra weight on babies. This extra weight on mother is usually difficult to lose and is usually the culprit for feeling pressure on the lungs while trying to take a deep breath.

Grains that have been ground are very hard on the thyroid and have a chemical effect on the brain that regulates emotion.

Baby Blues or Post Partum Depression are more frequent in women who eat ground grains and sugar. If a woman doesn't have extra weight to lose, from eating sugar or flour, than she doesn't have to work at losing it later which greatly helps ones self-esteem.

Yeast infections are fed by sugar, milk, flour and yeast (like that found in bread).

The cervix is affected by flour, making for longer labors by significantly slowing progress of cervical dilation causing labors to be much longer. The only women in my career who have had 14 plus hour labors, are the ones who refused to give up flour in their diet.

Acceptable Replacements
Whole Grains
Cracked Grains
Rolled Grains
Steel Cut Grains

NO MICROWAVE using a microwave to warm (or cook) food interferes with the electrical impulse within the human body. The heart, brain, nervous system, immune system and muscles can all be affected by the use of a microwave. In Sara Shannon's book, "Diet for the Atomic Age", she shows studies on the low levels of radiation and the serious effects on mothers and on the unborn child.

In 1970, when microwaves were first introduced into the United States the miscarriage rate was at 1 in every 40 pregnancies and by 1995 the miscarriage rate climbed much higher to 1 in every 4 pregnancies. During this same period the rate of heart disease and cancer also escalated in America, maybe it's coincidence or a variety of other negative lifestyle changes our society has made, but it's not worth the risk. Heating any fruit or vegetable kills 30% of the friendly bacteria and enzymes so eating a diet that consists of a high amount of raw vegetables and fruits, is very important for good digestive health. At least 50% of the vegetables and 70% of fruit should be eaten in a raw state.

Acceptable Replacements
Conventionally Cooked vegetables and fruits
Steamed vegetables and fruits
Raw Vegetables and Fruits

NO ACIDIC FOODS Citrus, coffee, tomato, cocoa etc., these foods cause digestive problems, bind the filtering system (kidneys, liver, and spleen), and lay foundation for arthritis, gout, and joint problems. Many of these problems have become common in our modern society and not only in adults, but in babies and small children.

There is not a problem with a few tomatoes on a salad or as a garnish, but they need to be eaten very sparingly. Low acid variety tomatoes would be acceptable if eaten sparingly.

Human pH should be between 5.5 and 6.5, which is slightly acidic. If our bodies are too alkaline then there are not enough acids to break down the foods in our diet, then adding in a small amount of acids can be helpful. If our bodies are too acidic than it can cause heartburn, indigestion, and achy joints. If this is the case then the acids in ones diet should be cut back or completely left out. The pH should be monitored throughout pregnancy and can be monitored by using urine strips, which can be found online or in most pharmacies.

Acceptable Replacements
Choose Less Acidic Foods
The acid in some foods can be neutralized by adding a little baking soda.

NO HEAT PRODUCING FOODS Cayenne, jalapeno, chili, salsa, curry, etc. These foods can cause inflammatory conditions such as headaches, joint pain, nosebleeds, excessive uterine bleeding, frustration, irritability, anger, hot flashes, and reddish complexions. Even though chili peppers are a common herbal supplement, their use should be limited in people who suffer any of the afore mentioned conditions. Cayenne, if taken in small amounts can help to slow bleeding, but if taken long term it can cause an inflammatory problem to build. There is usually 50% more bleeding in women who eat heat producing foods and also sugar. I am far more serious about restricting heat producing foods in women who show a tendency to bleed (nosebleeds, vaginal bleeding, bruising, bleeding when flossing or brushing teeth, have reddish complexions or have red hair).

Acceptable Replacements
Sweet or Mild Peppers
Mild, non-heat producing spices

NO PORK or PROCESSED MEATS Hot dogs, lunch meats, sausage, bacon, etc. It takes four hours for your body to digest fish or fowl, eight hours to digest beef and fourteen hours to digest pork. Any substance that stays in the body for fourteen hours starts to turn toxic and feeds poisons back into the body. Pork is also well known for parasites and infections, earning its claim to fame as "un-clean". Processed meats have a host of bacteria and to combat the high amounts of bacteria, companies add chemicals. These processed meats are usually made with poor grade meat, have additives, preservatives, and are also cured using nitrates. If it doesn't look like meat and looks as if it has been chopped, pressed, or altered stay away from it during pregnancy.

Acceptable Replacements
Beef
Fowl (turkey, chicken, duck etc)
Fish (ocean or freshwater fish)
Wild game (except wild boar)

NO SOY Tofu, soybeans, soymilk, or any soy product. Soy is high in estrogen and is sold in most nutritional centers for menopause. There is enough estrogen in eight ounces of soymilk, to relieve menopausal symptoms in many middle-aged women. This means there is too much for most other aged females or males of any age.

Estrogen is a wonderful hormone and definitely has its place in health, but during pregnancy the primary hormone should be progesterone. Progesterone is the hormone responsible for relaxing the muscles and uterus. The intake of soy during pregnancy increases estrogen, which causes contracting of the muscles including the uterus. From the first day a woman starts her period, to the day of ovulation estrogen is the primary hormone, and from the day of ovulation up until her period, (or days prior to delivery) the primary hormone is progesterone.

Exception: The only time I would suggest the use of soy milk during pregnancy is the last week before a woman's estimated due date. If she has a history of failing to go into labor, or has not had any Braxton-Hicks contractions. Braxton-Hicks show the body is producing estrogen and is preparing for labor.

Seasonings such as soy sauce, in small amounts, are fine if kept at a minimum and not used daily.

NO FRIED FOODS and WATCH THOSE FATS No vegetable oil, corn oil, cottonseed oil, canola oil etc. Any time there is a problem with the liver the recommendation for most is to stop eating fried or greasy foods. It should stand to reason that if you are trying to avoid a liver problem, that the recommendation would be the same. The liver is a primary part of the filtering system, and in our modern society the liver is seriously compromised with the various bacterial and viral infections we come in contact with. When you add in all the fried, greasy foods we eat it starts to take a toll on our liver.

Acceptable Alternatives
Bake
Roast
Broil
Boil
Steam
Stir-Fry using a very small amount of olive oil (sparingly)
Any type of Olive Oil (extra virgin, virgin, or light)
Raw Coconut oil
Butter (used sparingly and only if there are no problems with cholesterol)

Meal Time

Breakfast is an important opportunity to cleanse and open the channels of elimination. Hot, whole grains, such as cracked wheat, multi grain, or oatmeal, and a low acid fruit can help to assist in the cleansing process. If signs of a lowered blood sugar level such as nausea, vomiting, headaches, dizziness, shakiness, and/or mood swings occur after a meal than eggs or any other acceptable source of protein should be added to the meal. Protein helps to balance blood sugar levels.

NOTE: A high protein breakfast without a grain is acceptable, but the grains and fruits need to be added in throughout the day.

Lunch and Dinner are the time to build strength and energy and should consist of animal protein. Animal protein provides a good source of amino acids for strong and healthy muscle, bone, and chemical balance of the brain. Animal proteins are things like meats, eggs and naturally aged block cheeses.

Vegetarians have a tendency toward prolapsed organs, which is dangerous during the delivery of a baby. Every organ in the body is held up by muscle, and the muscle helps to keep structure. If there is not adequate nutrition then the muscles weaken causing the organ(s) to slip down out of place.

Make sure that all meat comes from a reliable source and is cooked completely. Knowing where your food comes from is more important today than it was in years past, because of the ever-growing diseases such as bird flu, mad cow, muscle wasting, and West Nile.

NOTE: Protein drinks or any protein supplement containing, amino acid isolates should not be taken during pregnancy and should never be a replacement for animal protein.

Vegetables eating at least two large servings of every color of vegetable per week provides a good source of vitamins, minerals, enzymes, and antioxidants. Vegetables are "builders" and are an important part of daily nutrition.

Rule: A woman should eat two servings of meat and two servings of vegetables for every serving of fruit. In other words, we should build twice as often as we cleanse when we eat.

Corn should be eaten sparingly. I have never found any harmful effects on women who eat corn, but it does a good job of adding extra weight.

Potatoes should be eaten no more than twice per week because of the high starch content. The starch in potatoes add extra weight and have the same issues that breads cause, if not eaten in moderation. Sweet potatoes or yams can be eaten freely without causing problems during pregnancy.

Legumes (plants with seeds in pods like beans, and peas) combined with an animal protein compliment each other and are a perfect protein, during pregnancy. Legumes are a good replacement for the starchy potato.

Leafy greens like lettuce, spinach, kale etc. give fiber for proper elimination and are blood builders due to their iron and vitamin K content. Leafy greens are helpful during pregnancy due to the high quality and volume of blood that is needed.

NOTE: Leafy greens should be eaten sparingly if there is thick blood or high blood pressure while they should be eaten more liberally by anyone with anemia or low blood pressure.

Water (from a clean source) helps to prevent low blood pressure, dehydration, constipation, sinus, and urinary tract infections and should be ingested throughout the day. I recommend 1 quart per 40 pounds of body weight be consumed, per day.

~~~~~A Short Story~~~~~

There was a woman of whom I assisted during the birth of her second baby. While she was pregnant with her third baby I moved out of state and gave her the option of having me travel for the birth of the baby or get a new birth attendant. She said that it would be worth having me travel because she did not want any other birth attendant. When I asked her "Why?" she said, "My first birth attendant told me that it didn't matter what I ate, just eat! Big babies are healthy babies!" Her first baby was over nine pounds and she labored for about 36 hours. Since she had been following the diet and supplement program she had a six and a half pound baby with only six hours of labor. She did not want to change anything. How could I resist? I made it back to deliver her little girl. Her baby weighed six pounds and her labor was only four hours long.

This woman is one of many who have seen the changes a healthy diet can bring. Most of our women would agree that it is worth the self discipline this diet takes because they are much healthier and feel better than they have ever felt. Many of the women that start on this diet not only use it during their pregnancies, but they make it a permanent lifestyle change. I was told by someone I highly respect "No diet is a good diet unless it can be used long term. If it is going to throw the body out of balance if used too long then it is not good for short term either." I have to agree.

Foods to Avoid

Sweeteners
    White Sugar
    Brown Sugar
    Raw Sugar
    Powdered or Confectioners Sugar
    Aspartame
    Sucralose or any other artificial sweeteners
    Carbonation (anything with a bubble)
(*Continued*)

Dairy
- Milk
- Cream
- Half & Half
- Whipped Cream
- Ice Cream
- Cream Cheese
- Cottage Cheese
- Sour Cream
- Yogurt
- Buttermilk

High acid foods
- Coffee
- Tomatoes
- Oranges
- Pineapple
- Lemons
- Limes
- All citrus

Heat producing foods
- Cayenne
- Jalapeno
- Salsa
- Habanera
- Curry
- Red Chili Peppers

Pork & Processed Meats
- Bacon
- Ham
- Sausage
- Pork Chops
- Pork Loins
- Lunchmeats
- Hot Dogs
- Bologna

Soy
- Soy Milk
- Soy Beans
- Tofu
- Soy Flour

Grains
- Breads
- White Flour
- Whole Wheat Flour
- Rice Flour
- Barley Flour
- Oat Flour
- Rye Flour
- Spelt or Sprouted-grain Flour
- Pasta
- Couscous

    Crackers
    Tortillas
    Cookies
    Cakes
    Pastries
Fats
    Fried Foods
    Vegetable Oils
    Canola Oil
    Lard
    Shortening
    Margarine

Never use a microwave. Not even to thaw, re-heat or defrost.

Foods to Eat Sparingly

    Potatoes
    Corn
    Shellfish
    White Rice
    Butter
    Soy Sauce

Foods to Eat Freely

Liquids
    Water
    Herbal Teas
    100% Low Acid Fruit Juices
Whole grains
    Cracked Wheat
    Pearl Barley
    Brown Rice
    Wild Rice
    Rolled Oats
    Steel Cut Oats
    Quinoa
    Amaranth
    Millet
Legumes
    Beans
    Peas
    Peanuts
    Green Beans
    Nut Butters
Hard (Block) Cheeses
    Cheddar
    Mozzarella
    American (*Continued*)

Swiss
Parmesan
Fruits
All non-acidic fruits
Vegetables
All with the exception potatoes
Meats
Beef
Poultry (Chicken, turkey, duck, pheasant etc)
Fish (ocean and fresh water fish)
Wild Game (Elk, deer, goose, etc)
Sweeteners
Honey
Stevia
Agave
Pure Maple Syrup
Molasses

~~~~~A Short Story~~~~~

Most of my children were born and raised with homebirth. Though my 17-year old son had been primarily home schooled, he did attend public school through high school. One day while in health class his teacher started teaching the class about pregnancy and what to expect. She told about weight gain expectations and my son raised his hand and told her, "That is only if they are eating breads, potatoes, carbonation and sugar. Excess weight is not expected if the proper foods are eaten." She listened and then continued on with her lecture. She started to talk about morning sickness being an acceptable part of pregnancy and he again raised his hand and politely told her, "Morning sickness has reasons such as liver or bowel problems or milk consumption and if those things are taken care of then there is no morning sickness". The teacher's lecture and my son's comments on pregnancy continued on throughout the class and finally the bell rang. The teacher said, "Class dismissed, except Mr. Young, would you please stay so I can talk to you?" He figured he was in trouble, but when the classroom cleared she walked over to him and asked, "Where did you learn so much about pregnancy?" He replied, "My mom delivers babies and I was home schooled. Did I do something wrong?" She replied, "No, my daughter is pregnant and we need some answers." The 17-year old boy sat in class after hours and answered questions for his teacher. He is a very bright young man, and I never thought he was listening, shame on me.

~~~~~A Short Story~~~~~

I had a client that insisted she was following dietary instructions. She never brought her husband to appointments, she said he had to work and could not make it. I had questions about her and she always had glucose in her urine, but would state it was from eating fruit or drinking juice. She gained a lot of weight, but insisted she had lost so much weight before she got on the program that her body was "regulating" and everything was fine.

The day came for the birth and she cried, screamed and wailed with every contraction. I spoke privately with her husband who told me she would not allow him to attend visits and he knew nothing about the diet she was supposed to be following. He told me that all she ate was sugar and that she had never changed her diet. He said, "In fact, she has had nothing to eat in the last 24 hours except a pan full of brownies and a gallon of orange juice." Shortly afterwards, she reached transition. She pushed the baby out in a reasonable time (this was not her first baby) and as soon as her baby was born she began to hemorrhage. We applied, cervical and low uterine pressure, ice packs, along with homeopathics and shepherd's purse tea to stop the bleeding. Her blood pressure was low, but not dangerously low. A few minutes later, she started asking to breastfeed her baby and from a lying position baby was latched on with some assistance. I headed to the other room to take care of other things and within minutes my assistant screamed that the mother was lying on top of the baby. When I got there, the assistant was in the process of rolling the mother over and retrieving baby. The husband stated she had done this same thing during her last delivery. It took us hours to stabilize this woman and finally felt that she was stable enough for us to leave. Before I left I gave special instructions for her to eat foods that would build her blood levels back and that her diet should be high in proteins and green vegetables. As I reached the edge of town I decided to give this family a call in case I needed to return and found that she was refusing to eat anything except chocolate covered strawberries.

This behavior is not uncommon for women who are sugar addicts. It is frightening and very dangerous for both mother and child. I did the recheck and also called and spoke to her and her husband several times after the birth of their baby. I then met with her for her six week checkup, at which she and baby were both doing fine. I did tell her she should not do another home birth, that she did not meet the qualifications for a low-risk birth. Two years later I heard she was pregnant again and she did go to the hospital to have her child, which was the best for all concerned. No one should risk the safety of a mother or child for the desire of a home birth.

~~~~~A Short Story~~~~~

When I think of vegetarians and birth it brings to mind an experience where the client was a woman who was a devout vegetarian. We talked about the diet and the fact that such a high percentage of people who do not eat meats tend to suffer from prolapsed internal organs due to lack of amino acids. She talked about her studies, and she convinced me that she had studied hard and knew all the right things to eat to fulfill all of the amino acids her body would need during pregnancy as well as labor and delivery and she and baby would be alright.

Throughout her pregnancy, I had no complaints about weight gain, urine tests, or vitals as everything checked good. She looked like a model, absolutely beautiful. The day of the delivery came, she had a long and difficult labor. Finally baby was descending down the birth canal and suddenly the reality of it all came forward. As the woman pushed, her vagina rolled outward ahead of the baby, a condition known as vaginal vault prolapse. I held the vagina up and in with the left hand and gave support to hold it into place as baby was birthed with the right hand. Considering everything, the push phase went rather quickly (too quickly to allow for a transport).

When baby was born, she was delivered out of naturally warm (98 degree) mother and baby had ice-cold hands and feet that were white from lack of circulation. A condition known as cyanosis, where there is inadequate oxygen in the body to circulate to the extremities causing, white in severe cases, usually blue coloring in the hands and feet. Baby was immediately given oxygen and measures were taken to stabilize her condition.

As I looked back over this incident, I believe that this situation could have been avoided had the mother had proper protein. Since that time, I have refused clients who will not eat meat, eggs or gelatin. Not that complications always arise, they are just more prone to happen and I feel they should be in a place where they are better equipped to handle emergencies.

~3~
SUPPLEMENTS

In this section, I explain the supplements we use during pregnancy, the usual amounts, what to expect and a general basic on how to adjust amounts. Remember that each woman's body is different and each woman needs to exercise her own personal responsibility, listen to her body and adjust amounts for the best outcome possible.

Prenatal tea, yester-year and today
For centuries, the cornerstone of a healthy pregnancy was considered to be a good prenatal tea. This tea was to include the herbs that were historically used to prepare a woman's body for a lower risk birth. Years gone by, midwives would generally recommend a prenatal tea that included the leaves of the red raspberry plant along with alfalfa, comfrey and nettle leaves as well as lobelia. Depending on the needs of the ladies in a given area a midwife would alter the recipe to fit her patient's needs. The tea would be made into a strong concoction with between 1 and 1½ quarts per day consumed. It could be consumed hot, warm or cold and was generally sweetened with a little honey.

The old-school midwives would have this type of logic:
Red Raspberry leaves were to strengthen and tonify the uterus and female organs without adding a hormone. Unlike most 'female supporting' herbs the raspberry leaves did not have, or stimulate the production of, estrogen nor progesterone. History had shown the ladies who consumed the raspberry tea tended to have a stronger uterus that performed more efficiently. This part of the tea would make up the largest percentage, about 40-50% of the total combination.

Alfalfa leaves were high in amino acids, Vitamins E, C, K as well as iron. Preventing low blood pressure and anemia while giving strength and providing antioxidants. It was also believed to prevent excess bleeding.

Nettle leaves were historically used to cleanse the liver and kidneys to prevent toxemia and kidney problems. It also had historical uses as a respiratory support during a time when respiratory issues claimed many lives. Not only did they want to avoid the liver and kidney issues but wanted to support the respiratory system in both mother and child. The chain reaction would be to avoid problems associated such as water retention, arthritis, gout, sciatica, bladder infections, asthma, bronchitis, pneumonia, laryngitis and coughs. Above and beyond these wonderful attributes it also got credited for preventing uterine hemorrhages and excessive menstrual bleeding making it a staple for pregnancy and women's health in general.

Comfrey leaves were found to strengthen the integrity of all muscle, bone, ligaments and connective tissue in the body as well as encourage healing to injured areas. It was found that women who would drink comfrey in their tea had much thicker amniotic sacs which lessened the chances of premature rupture of membranes. It did increase the chances of babies being born 'in the cull'. (Being born in the cull means to be born in the sac.) Years back this was believed to be a 'sacred child' or a 'miracle birth'. I, personally, consider it a complication if one does not have an experienced birth attendant to rupture the sac as there is a lot more pressure if the sac is intact during the birth process. It also increases the chances of pulling the placenta away from the uterus during the birth.

Lobelia was known as a 'self thinking' herb. If a practitioner did not know or understand the problem then lobelia was prone to bring the problem to surface to be identified. The lobelia was used in very small amounts to assist in ridding the body of infections of all types. Too much would induce vomiting but small amounts were used for everything from venoms, to bacterial, to viral infections and for 'when in doubt' situations. It is also a muscle relaxant that helped prevent miscarriages and calm uterine contractions without a hormone imbalance.

This combination was generally put into a mix of leaves consisting of about three parts Red Raspberry leaves, one part each Alfalfa, Nettle and Comfrey leaves with 1/8 part Lobelia herb. The amounts would vary depending on the midwife, the culture, geographical locations and availability of herbs. However, most midwives back in the day would recommend a tea similar to this one in order to prevent problems associated with pregnancy and birth. Note: The term "parts" means to use equal size measurements, whether it be cups, spoons or more. So if a person wants to make up a small batch for just a few days they would use a tablespoon for parts. If they are wanting to do enough for weeks then they would use a cup. If a batch were being made for several ladies, or pregnancies then they could possibly use pounds but this would be a very large batch. As a rule, a woman would use about 2 lbs total of prenatal tea during one pregnancy.

Today the basic herbs remain. Again, there are variances depending on the education and experience of the midwife. Each has their own reasons for doing things the way they do, whether it is based on education and experience or on misinformation and fear. A little questioning will bring to surface the reasons for recommending what one does.

The medical profession rarely recommends the use of herbs. Not, necessarily, because they have reason to dislike them but usually because they have not been educated to the value of them. The most common response I hear is "We know the herbs are doing something, we just don't know what kind of interaction they are going to have with the meds we are giving." They are correct. The herbs are doing something and their training is in the meds and they are not taught to understand the interactions.... Therefore it is best to err on the side of caution by leaving out the herbs that they do not understand.

Today things have changed. Many herbs are brought under scrutiny by the medical and political professions for a variety of reasons. Is it money? Partly. Is it control? Maybe. Is it from not being educated? To a point. Whatever the suspicions, the facts remain, some herbs are not approved through the government for human consumption. We always abide by the laws of our land and therefore we do not recommend herbs that are outlawed for whatever reason. If we are not happy with the laws, then they can be changed with enough effort. However, we do our best to abide by them until they are.

Disclaimer: Current laws do not allow the recommendation of Comfrey and, sometimes, Lobelia. To choose to use these herbs is done so at your own risk and the author assumes no responsibility for such actions.

With all this taken into consideration, there are new prenatal teas formulated by a variety of people and companies with different schools of thought. As for me? I remain with the old school. I liked their reasoning years back and it is the formula I used during my own last few pregnancies (and would use if I ever got pregnant again). It is the one I have seen results with in many clients years back. It has been used in our family so long we consider it a family recipe. Currently, it is unlawful to recommend Comfrey for human consumption throughout the United States. Some states have passed similar laws regarding lobelia. Therefore, I recommend one of the adapted versions (*Recipes on next page*)

Modern Prenatal Tea
4 parts Red Raspberry Leaves
1 part Alfalfa Leaves
1 part Nettle Leaves
Recommendation being a strong tea at 4 cups per day from as early as possible in the pregnancy (and even before conception would be a nice idea!) until baby is 6 weeks old. If there are going to be pregnancies close together, then the prenatal tea can be used on an ongoing basis. If a woman does not start on the tea until late in the pregnancy then she would drink more because she has less time to get her body prepared for the birth.

Modern Prenatal Tea II
4 parts Red Raspberry Leaf
1 part Licorice root
This one works well for women who do not like the taste of alfalfa and are eating plenty of greens. The licorice assists in helping to regulate blood sugar levels and to keep the blood pressure from dropping while still supporting the uterus. This tea is prepared and consumed the same as the regular Modern Prenatal Tea.

Pros and cons to the changes:
Comfrey: One of the changes that came with dropping the comfrey is there are more pre-term births and more frequent premature rupture of membranes. Due to the fact the comfrey added more elasticity into the sac as well as giving it more integrity and a thicker texture. For this same reason, drinking the comfrey can also increase the chances of baby being born in the cull. This may sound like a magical and sacred deal but it is a much more difficult labor because the amniotic fluid is birthed with the baby and it is a more difficult birth to pass all this in the birth canal at the same time. Along with this comes the increased chances of a uterine hemorrhage. Why? Well, the sac is attached to the placenta and if the baby pulls the sac out of the mother while being born the placenta is also being pulled. As the placenta is being pulled away from the uterine wall there is almost always a hemorrhage. If the birth attendant is willing, and able, to break the water before the baby descends into the birth canal the chances are much better of a low risk delivery. If a woman finds herself alone, for whatever reason, then it is almost impossible for her to break her own water. I, personally, cut back on the amount of comfrey I used in my own last pregnancy because of these same issues and I was working towards a shorter birth time and had no intentions of having a labor long enough to allow another professional time to get there. Being without an experienced birth attendant to rupture the membranes, we did not want to risk the chances of a baby born in the sac. The lady I had with me was familiar with how I worked, had several children of her own but had limited actual birth experience. She did know how to follow instructions and was able to transport in the event of an emergency. We were less than one mile from the local hospital. Stopping the comfrey in the last trimester resulted in my water breaking prior to me being fully dilated, hours before labor.

Babies are immune from most things in their environment as long as the water is in tact. Once the membranes are ruptured, the baby is exposed to the microorganisms in the environment. Leaving the water in tact until mother is near or fully dilated is generally the better plan for baby. This was an advantage comfrey gave back in the day....keeping the sac intact until baby is ready to be born is a good thing. If the water has been broken for 24 hours the body begins to build infection and the mother-to-be needs to be watched very closely for signs of infection. This is done by monitoring her temperature and taking frequent urine tests. At any time there are even slightly elevated leukocytes or nitrites then she needs to be seen by a medical practitioner. If this is a home birth, she needs to be transported to a medical facility.

One of our ladies added 4 extra cups of comfrey tea, per day, to her program throughout the pregnancy. (She held this bit of information from me until the labor.) When doing an exam I could feel there was something unusual about her sac and I questioned it. She said her husband had told her to drink extra comfrey to insure the baby did not arrive early.... She had had another baby born at 36 weeks and their focal point was to hold baby in until it's due date. When she was fully dilated, I went to break her water and found that it was too strong for the plastic /disposable amni-hook to break. After trying 3 different hooks I finally reached for my surgical steel one. It broke the sac with ease. After the birth, we examined her placenta and sac, finding the sac was definitely the thickest I had ever seen and strong enough to have pulled the placenta away from the uterus, had she not had her water broken. Having this much pressure on a mother and child does not seem to be the better plan. All things in moderation.

Lobelia: Used for centuries as a remedy for respiratory issues and a muscle relaxant as well as to pull venoms and neutralize, or extract, organic poisons. Used to prevent miscarriages, sore muscles, treat snake or insect stings and rid depression. Used in very small amounts it was used for conditions such as asthma, muscle cramps, gastrointestinal cramps, uterine cramps and pre-term labor. Due to the alkaloid 'lobeline' contained, it was historically used to stop smoking. It was used for external treatment for bites and conditions such as staph and strep infections.

In larger amounts it was used for expelling the contents of the stomach. Great for food poisoning or over consumption, back in the day.

Due to the tendency to induce vomiting, if used in larger amounts, those who already suffered morning sickness found the lobelia to add to the vomiting. Vomiting itself can cause dilation or premature labor. If it is desired to use lobelia, most conditions can get similar results without taking it into the digestive tract and using it topically in a tincture of alcohol.

These days, we keep a bottle of the alcohol based extract (tends to be a little stronger, hence more effective than the vinegar) on hand for external use to add to the bath during labor or else rub into the areas where our mother-to-be is feeling the majority of her pains during labor. This is a win-win situation.

Our Family Prenatal Tea recipe is listed here...again, for educational reasons....this is the recipe I used for my last pregnancy (until the last month when the comfrey was dropped) and most immediate family members like this one.

Family Prenatal Tea recipe
4 parts Red Raspberry Leaves
1 part Licorice root, cut and sift
1 part Nettle leaves
1 part Comfrey Leaves
Strong tea at four cups per day from as early as possible in the pregnancy until baby is six weeks old. If there are going to be pregnancies close together, then the prenatal tea is used on an ongoing basis. I do not see the need for the alfalfa because we tend to eat lots of greens and beets and the alfalfa becomes a non-issue. We do tend to have low blood pressure which is assisted by the licorice root. This is an example of how things are altered to fit a given situation based on experience and knowledge.

We happen to live in a day and age which gives us advantages over other times in history. We have years of research into the value of specific vitamins, minerals, herbs, essential fatty acids and amino acids. Companies now provide products that were not available years ago. We have a transportation system that allows us to make use of products from around the world and have them brought right to our front door. We really live in a wonderful time for those reasons.

At this point we are including the supplement program I recommend for many of my ladies. The reader needs to understand I am not promoting any one specific company but give reference to some company names only so you can research the product and either use the ones I do or else find one comparable that you are comfortable with.

Supplements throughout Pregnancy

Beginning as soon after conception as possible.... Yes, it can be used prior to conception and between pregnancies.

Folic Acid plays a major role in cell division. Cell division is the process by which the cells divide and re-divide to form the baby from the initial egg and sperm cells. Without proper cell division there is an increased chance of birth defects. This is most important during the first trimester when the parts of baby are being formed. Folic acid also plays a role in the formation of hemoglobin, which is another important issue in pregnancy. Recommended amount 1 (one) .4mg (or 400 mcg) capsule per day.

Super Supplemental with Iron (Nature's Sunshine Products) is a multi-vitamin and mineral (MVM) combination that has always given us good results. Not only in pregnancy but in general for adults who have extra demands on their system. With our rapid growing methods our produce tends to be low in many of the nutrients that we would normally expect, so to supplement the diet we add in a high quality MVM. I have used this one for years and gotten results in a wide range of circumstances where there were high demands on a body, whether it be male or female, always an adult. The high B-complex supports the nervous system as well as providing energy. If taken too late in the day it will probably cause a sleepless night. When a good MVM is taken, there should be a notable change in the energy level. Suggested use is two tablets with breakfast and two with lunch. Light weight, or sensitive, women would need a little less. Maybe one or two morning and one lunch and always take with food in the stomach.

Note: After the birth I will suggest the husband take two of the Super Supplemental each morning for the next two weeks to ensure his strength while taking care of mother and child, usually while holding down a job. His body will have extra demands during this time and he will appreciate the added support.

Vitamin E (d-alpha) (any brand) 400 i.u. d-alpha is a natural vitamin E. We always use a natural source. Vitamin E assists the body in healing without scarring, assists in oxygen assimilation and is a powerful antioxidant assisting with immune support. Under most conditions one per day is plenty. There may be need for additional under certain circumstances. Vitamin E is an oil soluble vitamin, which means it is not broken down with water, so it is possible to overdose if a person takes too much for an extended period of time. Anything over 600 i.u. should be short term only. *(See miscarriage troubleshooting for more information)*

Prenatal tea is made by taking one teaspoon of the mixed leaves *(recipe prior in this section)* and put into one cup of boiling water (not microwaved). Let stand at least fifteen minutes and drink. Drink at least four cups per day. Can be made in larger amounts to be consumed throughout the day. Can be sweetened with honey and can be consumed warm or cold. Can this combination be taken in capsule form instead of in tea? Yes, it is generally not quite as effective but it runs a nice second place.

Add at the Beginning of the 25th Week

Granulated Soy Lecithin assists in forming the mucous lining around the heart, brain and lungs as well as other functions in the body. The use of lecithin, along with the rest of the program, is found to result in babies with a very high IQ, learning very rapidly. The purpose here is three fold. 1) To lessen the chances of low mood swings in our mother-to-be. 2) Increase the brain volume density to assist in baby staying into a vertex (head down) position. 3) Assist in baby's ability to take first breath easily. General recommendation is one tablespoon with a meal twice per day. It can be put in a pulped juice or sprinkled on oatmeal etc. Personally, I mix it with a glass of apricot juice and it is easy to drink. The intelligence is just a nice little side effect we get from the lecithin not our reason for taking it.

Calcium. I use a combination with four kinds of calcium that do not tend to build kidney or gall stones. The ingredients in this one include Calcium Phosphate, Calcium Citrate, Calcium Gluconate and Calcium Lactate as well as Phosphorus in the form of Calcium Phosphate and Magnesium in Magnesium Oxide and magnesium Carbonate forms. During pregnancy a woman requires more calcium because of the new little bones, muscle, tissue that are being built within her womb. Calcium is also a precursor to pain killing and blood clotting properties in the body. Extra calcium helps with the comfort during pregnancy as well as increasing pain tolerance during labor. Other nice attributes of taking it is the lessening of muscle cramps (Charlie horses) during pregnancy as well as working as a calmative. If she does not take supplemental calcium and is not getting adequate amounts in her diet then the baby will pull reserves from the mother's body, leaving her with deficiency symptoms. Signs of calcium deficiency include but are not limited to muscle cramps, bruising, any kind of bleeding (teeth, nose etc), rapid heart rate, insomnia, acid reflux, heartburn, anxiety and pain. Most expectant mothers will need about 1,200mg of calcium per day but those with extra needs (signs of deficiency) may need as much as 3,600mg (throughout the day with the largest dose taken before bed). When it starts making her tired during the day, it needs to be cut back. This usually takes about two weeks.

The best sign to tell if a calcium supplement is being assimilated is to take your resting heart rate. Take two tablespoons of the calcium, wait thirty minutes and take your resting heart rate again. If it is being assimilated then the heart rate should be lower than the rate prior to taking the calcium. Calcium products from a rock base (ie coral, bone meal, oyster shell, egg shell etc.) are less apt to break down to a molecular level therefore increasing the chances of causing gall or kidney stones and less apt to slow the heart rate. Due to the decreasing of the heart rate, it is best to take two tablespoons before bed which assists in a relaxing sleep as well as helping to set baby into a routine of going to sleep at night instead of having 'off hours'.

We have had evidence over and over that the blend of calcium I recommend is effective by waiting until a woman has reached a high point of pain and then give her four tablespoons of calcium. Within the next couple of contractions she will state that the sharp edge of the pain is diminished, sometimes to a point of heavy pressure. This is a big change that is seen within minutes but only with this type of calcium.

Colloidal Minerals (the bitter, unflavored, unsweetened ones are most effective) We are finding, over the last few years, more and more ladies are showing mineral deficiencies, even beyond the added mineral intake with the multi vitamin and mineral supplement. Adding the extra liquid minerals seems to lessen the number of symptoms ladies show. Posterior (aka slipped or prolapsed) cervix, irregular heart beat (on mother or child), excess sweating, nausea, dehydration, poor muscle tone, shortness of breath, backache and weakened immune system are some signs that can occur from a multi-mineral deficiency.

The stabilized mineral content in the human body (amniotic fluid, tears, blood etc) is identical to clean ocean water. Instead of using a lab formulated blend, it seems only natural to take the minerals in the same balance as nature itself intended. From an ancient sea bed (free of modern day contaminants), re-hydrated into a liquid form and then removing any solid sediment that could result in kidney or gall stones. One ounce per day is usually adequate for an expectant mother and is not too bad if mixed with juice to drink.

Add at the Beginning of the 35th Week

Evening Primrose Oil 1300 mg softgels (cold processed- any brand) contains essential fatty acids that are specially balanced for the female body. It is known for its ability to not only help with skin and cosmetic issues but PMS symptoms and hormone balance too. Historically, many cultures are deficient in essential fatty acids that lend to a tendency towards addictions, depression as well as slow dilation and effacement during labor. Often, but not always, it is found in lighted eyed, lighter skinned people of European ancestry. Another group the deficiency is found in would be Native Americans. These cultures are prone to have a higher incidence of long labors.

I personally do not like pain, not for myself nor for my clients. The better the pain tolerance and the more prepared the body, the better I like it. I like to see short labors in our ladies because we find there are fewer complications that way. Evening Primrose has a history of significantly shortening labors. If EPO is taken as a supplement during the last weeks of the pregnancy, the cervix is prone to soften and efface more readily, prior to the onset of labor. If the cervix is thin and pliable when labor begins then the labor is shorter than if the cervix is still thicker and firm.

The amount of Evening Primrose Oil varies from one lady to another.
1) If a woman has a history of long labors or is a first time mom then we start with 3 of the 1300mg soft gels 3 times per day. This gives the extra EFAs needed for more effective effacement and dilation.

2) If a woman has a history of 3-4 hour labors then 2 soft gels of EPO twice per day is generally enough. When 2-3 weeks prior to her due date, if the cervix has not shown significant softening and effacement then the amount is increased slightly to 2 soft gels 3 times per day. If the softening and ripening of the birth canal and cervix is going well, then leave the amounts.

3) If a mother has eaten no breads and has a history of labors shorter than 3 hours, then it is not a good idea to take the EPO supplement unless she is fully prepared to handle a very short labor. It works fine if it is a home birth with attendant nearby or she is very near to the birth center / hospital.

4) We have ladies who have made the unilateral decision to take extreme amounts, due to a long labor time previously. These amounts will run over 20 capsules per day, during the last week or two. We find these labors are generally less than ¼ the time of prior labors. This has obvious pros and cons to it.

I had one little gal who had a history of longer labors and wanted to make sure that she had a shorter one with the current pregnancy. She followed all instructions with diet and supplements. However, I found out near the end of the pregnancy that she had been taking 60 capsules per day of evening primrose oil for the last several weeks prior to the birth. Oh Goodness, I would never recommend those kinds of amounts! Well, it came time for the birth and her total labor time was about 10 minutes. If I had not been standing in the room when she started labor I would not have made it to the birth. *She* did not realize she was in labor until about the time the baby crowned.

This proves to have its pros and cons. Short labors are a heaven-send if everything is put together and the woman is with her birth attendant. There are fewer complications in short labors than in long ones. On the other hand, short labors do not give time to travel or make arrangements and run a higher risk of babies being born in route to the hospital or before the midwife arrives.

It is not advised to use the EPO to try to shorten a labor in spite of making bad food choices. The body needs to have balance and harmony to work properly. Personal responsibility is still the cornerstone to a positive birth experience.

Ground Ginger (bulk) is not an oral supplement but used in Ginger baths during the last 6 weeks of pregnancy. The ginger baths are used to increase circulation and generate elasticity into the perineum to prevent tearing at the birth. Add one tablespoon of ground ginger into a tub of bath water and soak for 30 minutes, once per day. There will be grit from the ginger so a rinse cycle will be needed. ☺ If there is any kind of irritation from the ginger baths then cut back on the amount to half. The ginger baths are especially important for first time moms and those with prior episiotomies or tears as these ladies are most prone to tear during a birth and the added elasticity is appreciated during that crowning.

Add at the beginning of week 39

Liquid Blue Cohosh causes the cervix to soften and efface. This, along with the EPO and diet, are responsible for the short labors. Blue Cohosh has been used for centuries for the purpose of 'silently' preparing the cervix for birth. This means the cervix will usually efface without the need for contractions. One dropper full in a cup of warm water two times per day, with meals, is usually sufficient.

Note: If you have a history of extremely short labors then this one should not be taken. Always, plan time to get to your place of choice to birth.

If too much is taken, it will result in an upset stomach with a few minutes after ingesting. Adjust accordingly.

Supplement recommendations are general recommendations. Each supplement is individualized to the needs of the mother. A woman is going to get out what she puts in. My intent is to give enough information that each mom can determine for herself how much to use, depending on her signs and symptoms. A little common sense and listening to your body and you should get the results you want. The choices are yours.

Notes_____

_____

_____

_____

_____

_____

~4~
KALA'S STORY

Growing up I always thought that I was special because I was born at home. As a small girl, I can remember my mom telling my brothers and I about how we came into this world. She told us of her pregnancies and labors. One of the most memorable stories is of my mom going into our yard and pulling up dandelion plants and blending them into her 'green drink'. I remember thinking that she must have been bit of a flower child back then, but now that I am older and have three babies of my own, her herbal concoctions are similar to what I use when I am pregnant. Her 'flower child' tendencies must have passed on to me.

At the age of 19, I was pregnant with my first baby. My husband Jori and I were so excited, it felt like I had been waiting my whole life to have my own babies to love. My sole priorities in life were to be a mommy and have a family. Now that my life goal was set into motion, I knew that I needed help and advice on how to have a baby "my own way". I needed to get prenatal care and decided to go to the local woman's health clinic, because this was where everyone else was going. After sitting in the waiting room for close to an hour, I finally got to meet with the doctor for an entire five minutes. I knew that this was not where I wanted to deliver my baby. My mom told me of a health food store in our town that was run by a midwife. We called and made an appointment with Donna Young. On the day of my first visit Jori and I walked into her quaint little herb shop, Donna walked out from the back and greeted us like she had known us for years. She was warm, gentle, compassionate, and a genius when it came to pregnancy, babies, and health. I knew at a young age that I wanted to have my babies at home just as my mom did. I knew right away I wanted Donna to guide me through my pregnancy.

I still remember how strict and scary Donna's diet and supplement regimen sounded. I trusted what she said and knew that if I wanted her to deliver my baby I would need to do what she recommended. Never in my life did I have to watch what I ate and I struggled immensely and I paid the price. During that first pregnancy my face never seemed blemish-free, I gained extra weight, felt out of shape, and my energy level was severely diminished. My husband would scold me and even teased about telling Donna if I ate something that I wasn't supposed to.

After a very long, hard, and intense labor it was time to push. I pushed for several hours and my baby was not coming. Her heart rate began to drop and we all knew we had to transport to the local hospital. She was born naturally with the help of the doctor's very forceful hands. I knew that she needed help, but as a midwife myself, I can't imagine inserting both of my hands into one of my girl's to pull a baby out. My body was traumatized and I was barely able to get out of bed for about a month. My spirit was totally wrecked. Once I recovered physically and emotionally, I knew that my next pregnancy I would strictly follow Donna's diet.

When I became pregnant again I faithfully followed diet and it showed. My skin was clear and radiant, and because I was so disciplined I felt strong and empowered. My second pregnancy came to an end on a beautiful September morning. I remember having contractions, but they weren't as painful as they were with my first, I was in control of these contractions and it was liberating. After about four hours of very light labor I called Donna and gave her the heads up on my progress. I told her there was no hurry. Donna said that she would shower and get ready, but a couple of contractions later I called her back, interrupting her shower, and told her it would be a good idea

Powerfully Pregnant

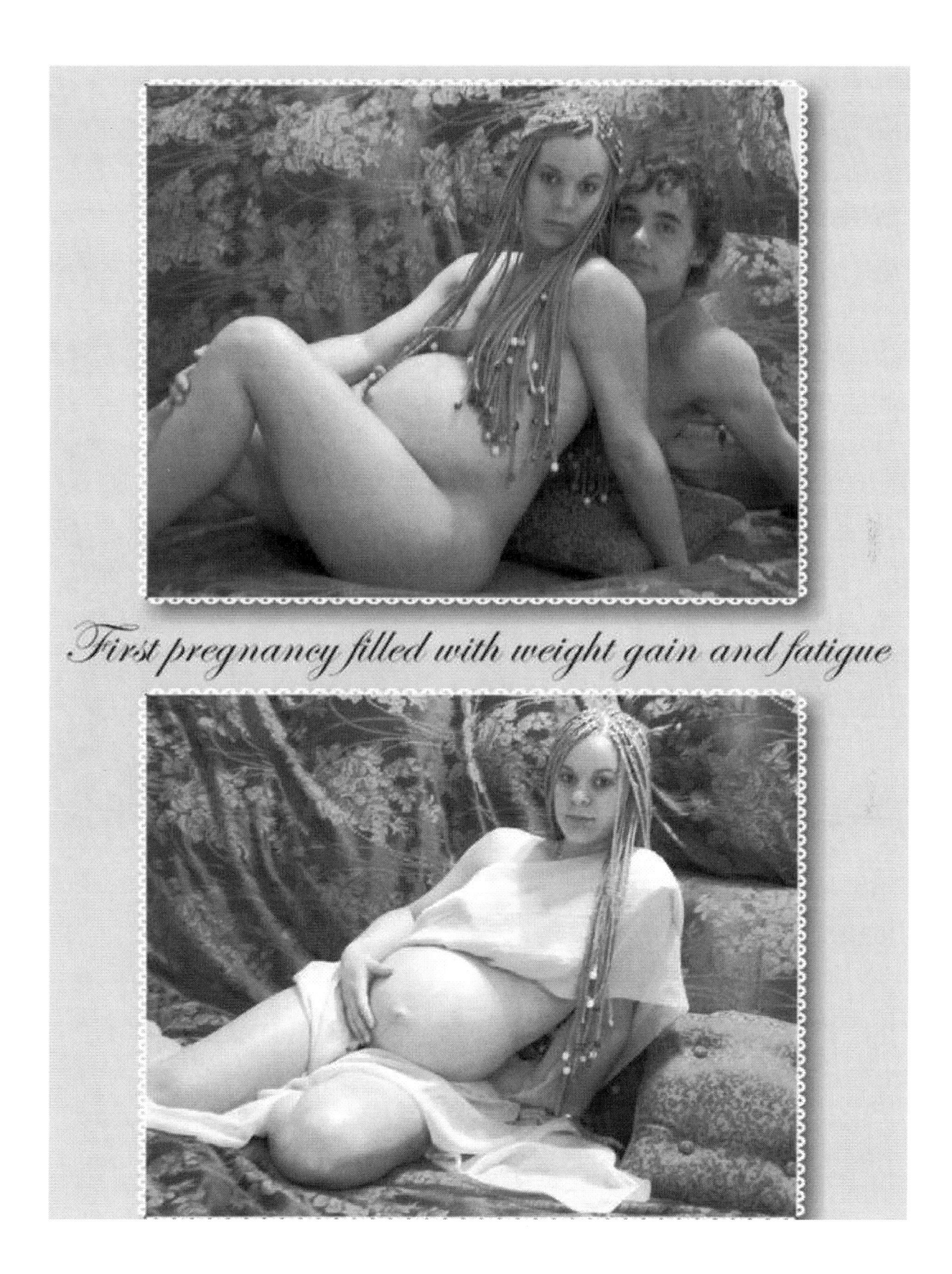

First pregnancy filled with weight gain and fatigue

Powerfully Pregnant

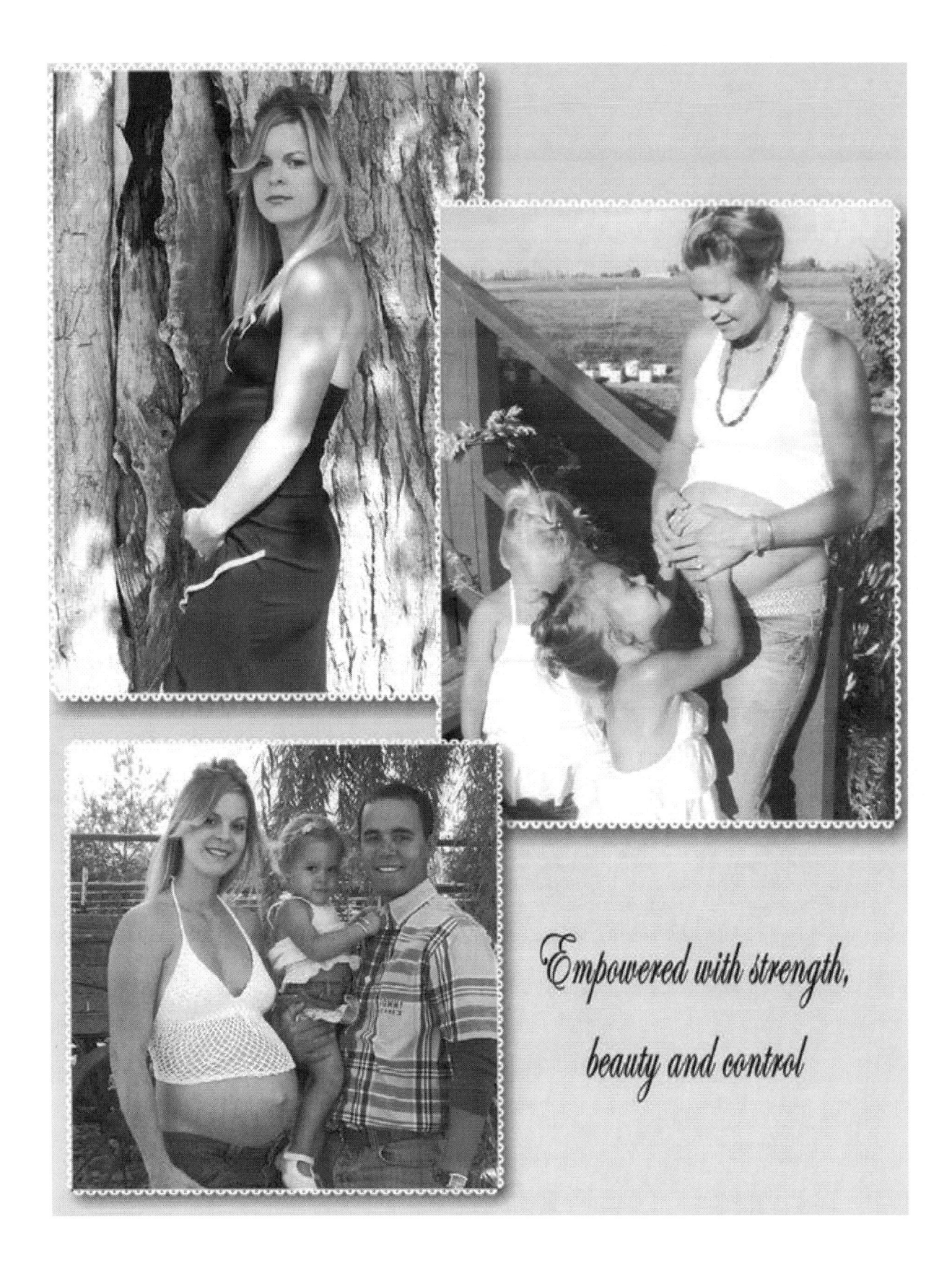

Empowered with strength, beauty and control

Powerfully Pregnant

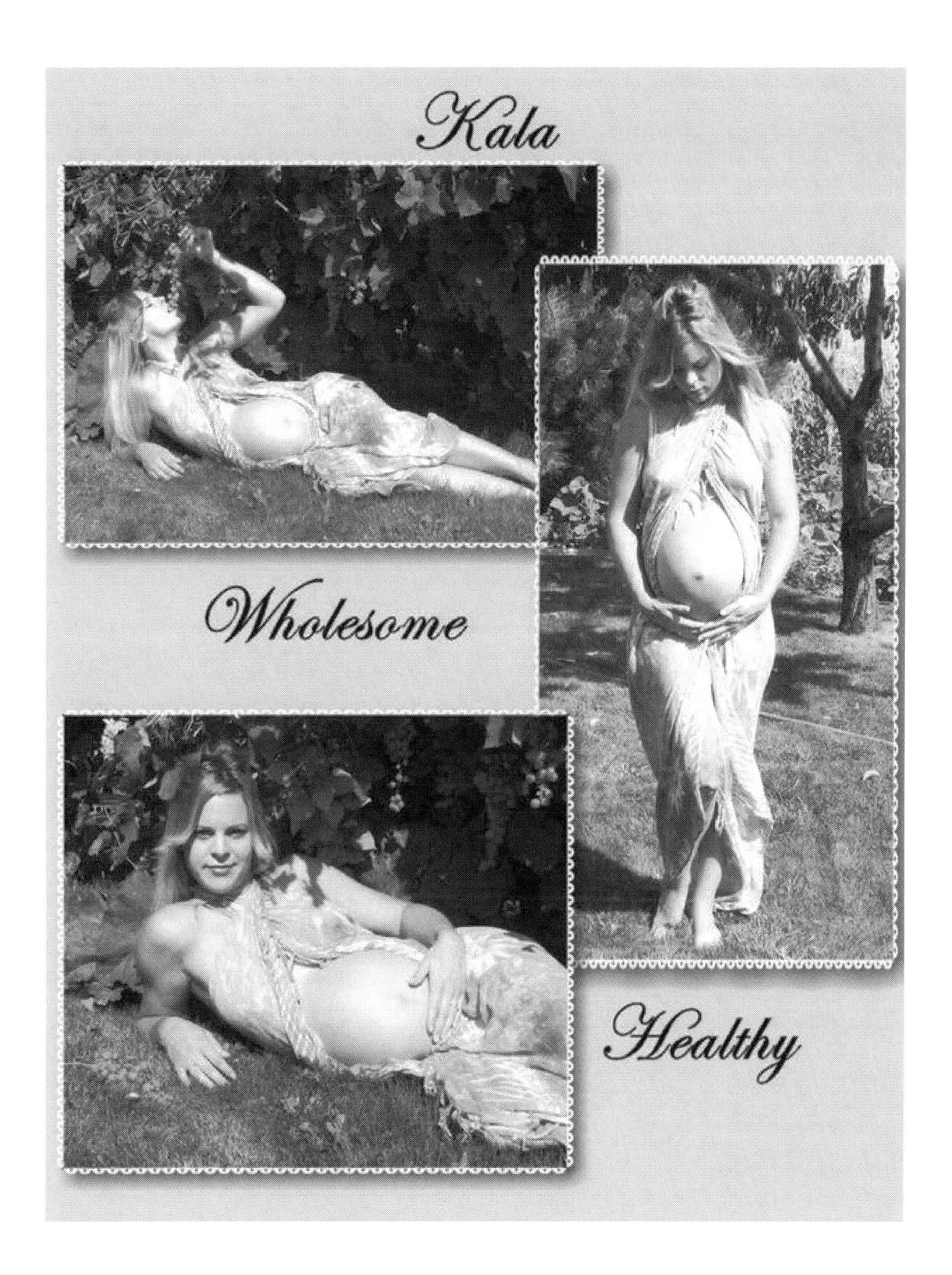

Kala

Wholesome

Healthy

for her to come over. Donna calmly arrived in about 10 minutes, she checked my cervix and it was time to have my baby. She broke my water as we smiled and joked through the contraction and the baby soon followed. What happened next transformed my life forever. Jada, my sweet little angel, came into this world pink as a rose and twice as beautiful. Her birth rejuvenated my soul. With five hours of labor and two pushes, I felt like there wasn't anything in this world I couldn't do.

Two years later, it was that time again; I was pregnant and ready for another sweet little soul to be a part of our family. I had revamped my kitchen and the way that I shopped and cooked, which made it much easier to abide by Donna's rules. In 2009, twelve days past my due date, on a much anticipated, July morning, I woke up at 7:00 a.m. I ate a big breakfast with two ounces of castor oil. A few hours later, my uterus began to tighten and relax in a rhythm typical of early labor. I was a busy mom of a two and four year old, so I didn't pay too much attention to the contractions. My philosophy is that if the pain doesn't stop you in your tracks, then you don't stop to worry about it. I began my morning chores and the instant that I felt my home was ready I called my mom, who lives about a half a mile away, to come over and braid my hair.

My mom arrived and with the very next contraction, I felt an intense urgency to call my husband home. My mom knew that we did not have long and there was no way we were going to braid my hair. I walked back to my bedroom and called Jori. He is a lineman for Idaho Power and was 90 feet in the air at the time fixing someone's power. I asked him to come home when he was finished. A few minutes later, literally, I called him back and said I changed my mind and he needed to come home to help deliver our baby, now! Donna had moved away and so we had two of my midwife friends, Connie and Lisa, attend the birth just in case something went wrong. About 20 minutes after I first called Jori, he walked in the door of our bedroom as I was having a contraction. I told him sternly that he better get in the shower. Two minutes later, he was out and had blue scrub pant bottoms on and a t-shirt. Still wet from his shower, he came to me, gently rubbed up against me, and calmly asked what he could do. I told him to put on gloves to see where the baby was. To his surprise he felt the baby's head as my water broke. At this point, Connie and Lisa walked in and I informed them in a calm, joking voice that, "The baby is coming right now". I don't think that they took me very seriously until they watched me bend over the side of my bed and push. Both of my hands were holding the baby's head in, to help prevent a tear and Jori told me to move my hands so he could catch our baby. I moved my hands and screeched, "Don't drop my baby". Looking back, I find it kind of funny that I told him not to drop our baby. Jori has the most caring and capable set of hands that I have ever known.

He slowly eased our baby into this world with the help of my one and only push. I turned around to look at my babe's face and slid down the side of my bed to sit on the floor. Jori handed me our sweet baby boy. He had gone from my nourishing womb to his daddy's gentle hands and back into my loving arms. There are no words to describe the divine bliss of this moment. As I lay my baby boy in my lap I snapped back into the reality of making sure all was well with my new little one and myself. He was a little bluish so I started to rub him with a dry towel to get him to "pink up". I then gave him some vitamin E, cayenne on the cord, and started with some blow-by oxygen. After I checked him out completely and knew he was healthy, I looked down at him and shouted in a joyful cry to Jori, "It's a boy"! We had wanted a baby boy so bad and he was finally here. My birth experience was better than I could have ever imagined. I am so blessed to be one of the few women today to have had the perfect birth experience. All I wanted to do was to educate and inspire other woman to have what I had.

Jordan's Birth

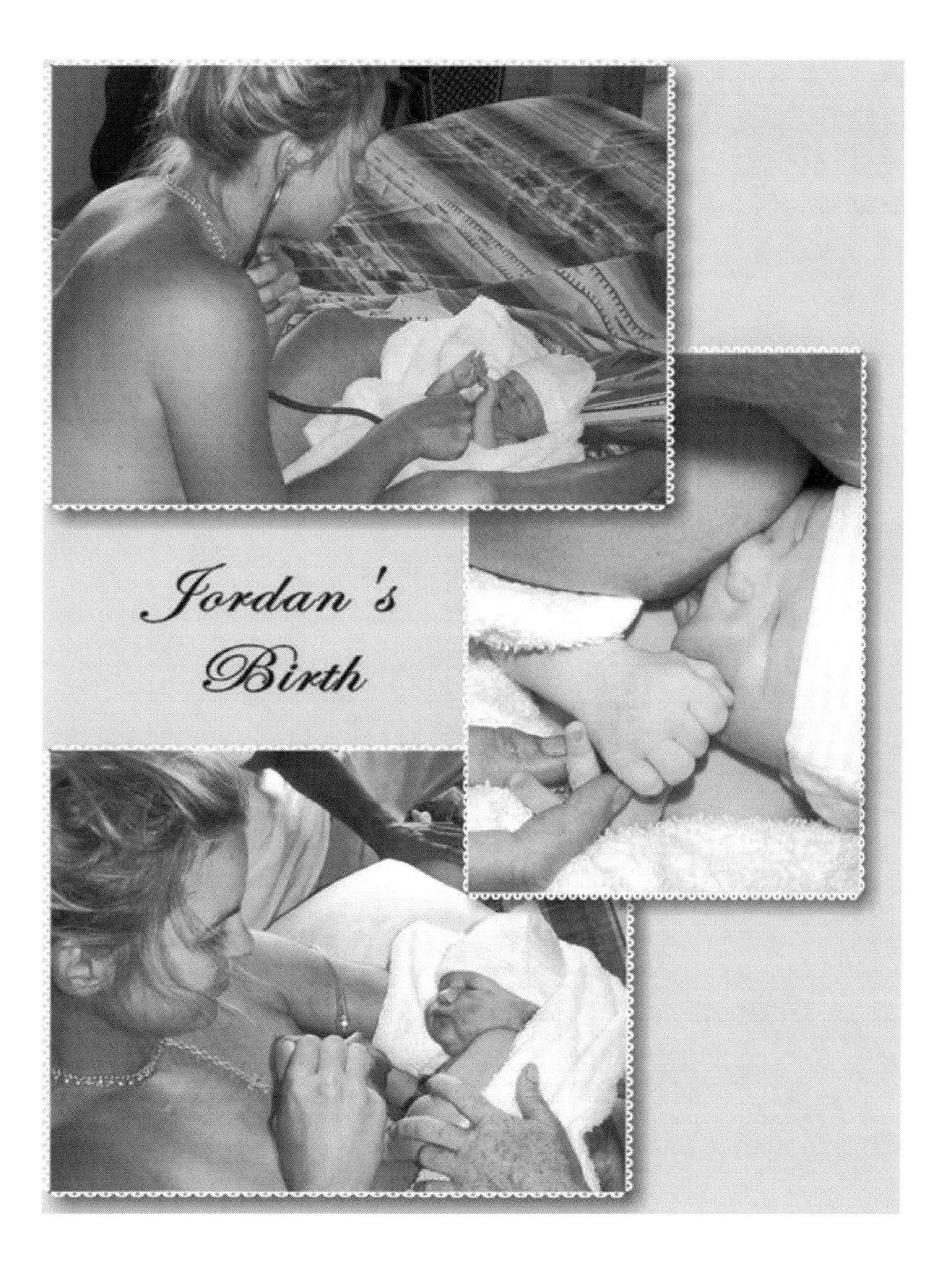

That Precious time after Jordan's Birth

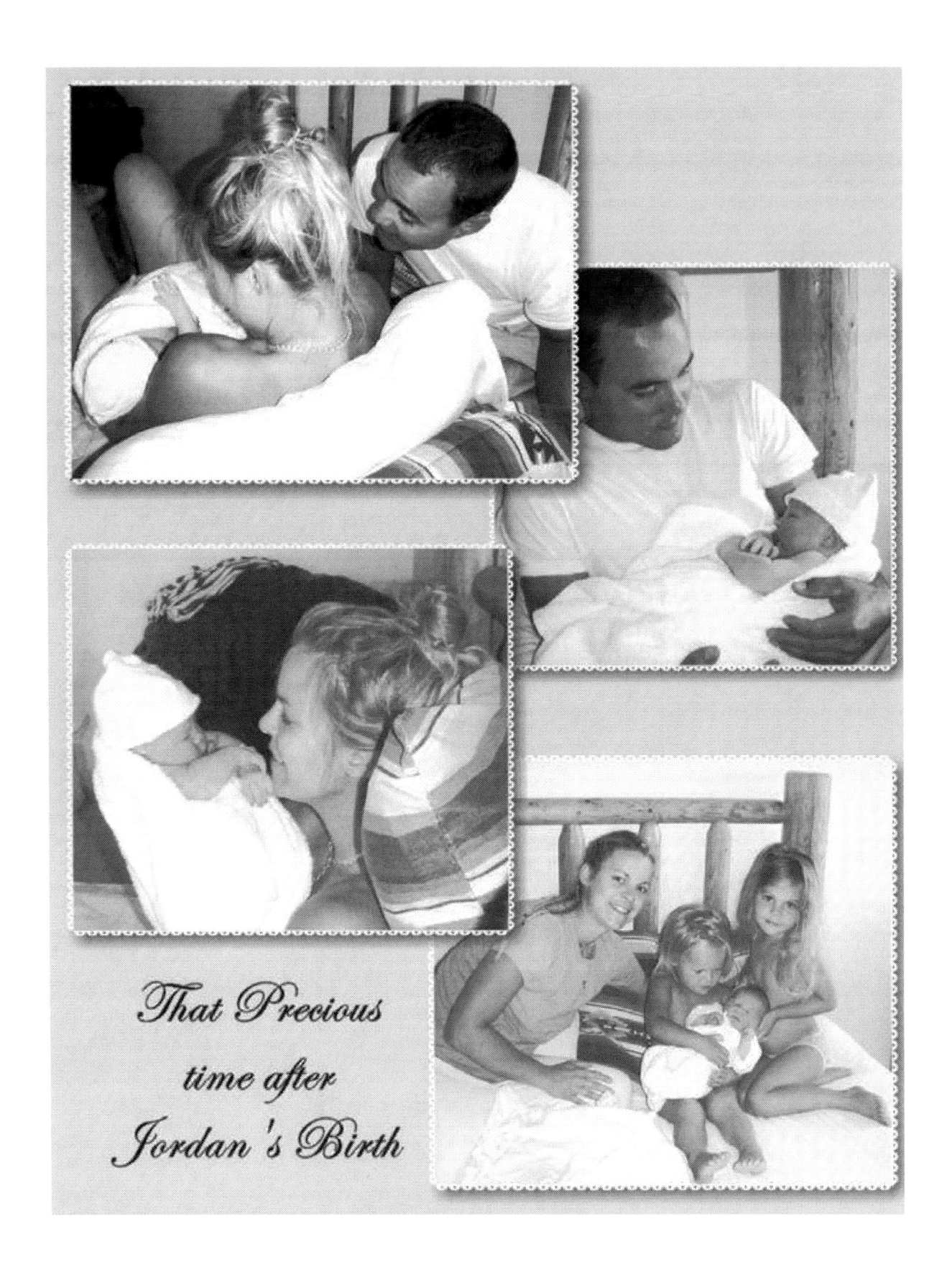

Powerfully Pregnant

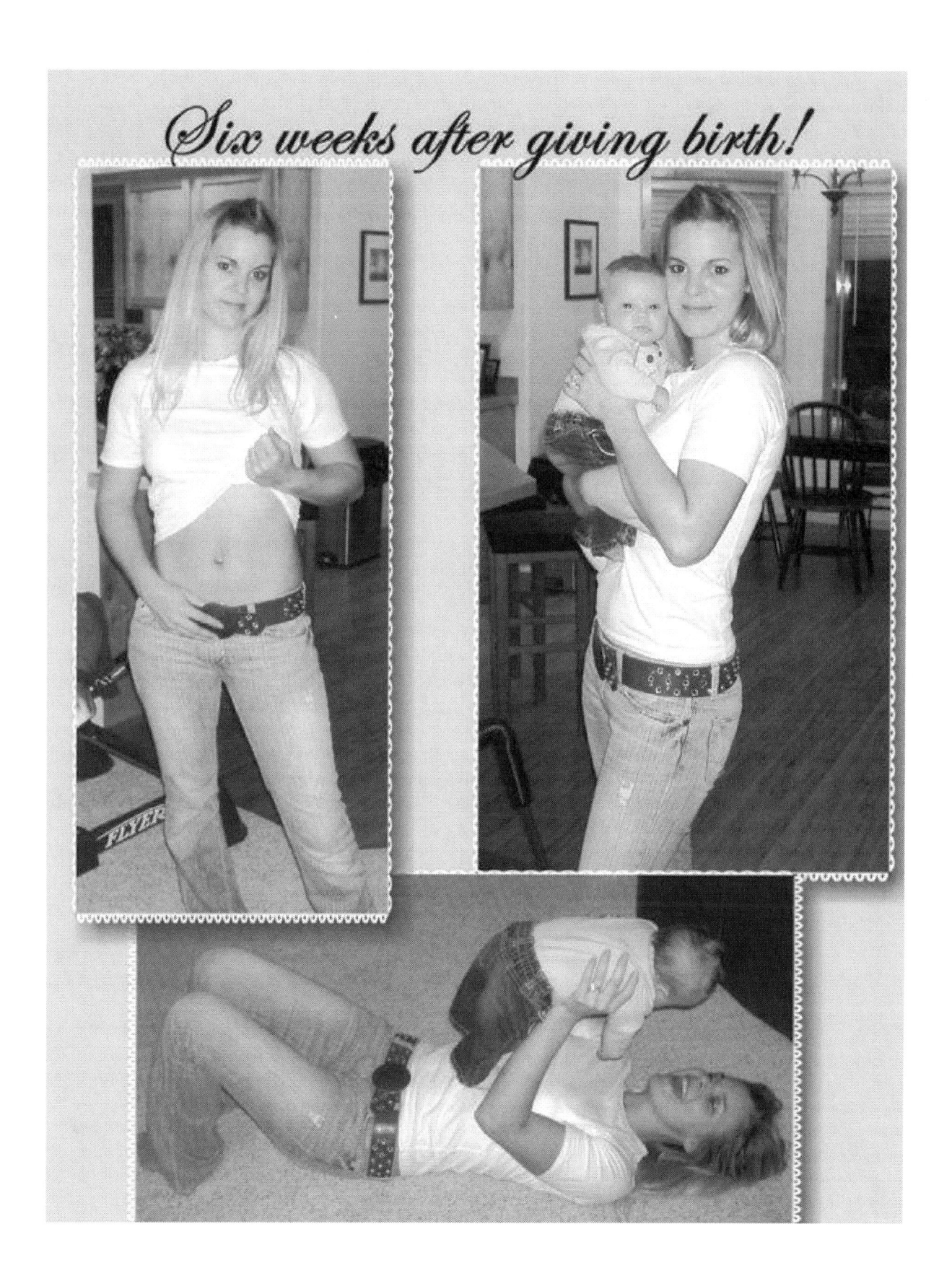

Six weeks after giving birth!

My midwifery career began after Shaila, my first baby girl, was born. I was 20 years old and began to apprentice alongside of Donna. I assisted as she delivered babies and I also helped with prenatal and postnatal care. The time came for Donna to shove me out on my own to deliver babies. She felt I was ready and I was confident that I could help mothers bring their babies into this world and gain the same empowerment that I had experienced with my births. She passed her clients in Idaho onto me and I began my journey as a midwife. I can remember the first baby I planned to deliver on my own so well. The call came in the middle of the night. Driving down my country road to Heidi's house, I can remember the anxious, tingly feeling I had over my entire body. I prayed a prayer that stuck with me for all my births to follow. It goes like this…. "Dear Lord, please guide my hands and my thoughts. Please allow me to think clearly and have the know-how to do what is right if a complication should arise. Be with my mom, my babe, and me. Keep us safe, healthy, and happy. In Jesus name I pray, Amen." This little prayer brings peace to the long drives. When I arrive at a birth, I have a comforting confidence that engulfs my thoughts. I feel calm and collected. I know my families appreciate this, because I've been told on many occasions that my peaceful demeanor is reassuring to a sometimes-stressful situation. I have Donna to thank for this. She is always calm and collected and even when complications arise her attitude stays this way. My first delivery on my own was beautiful and everything went perfect. I was on top of the world. I felt whole and complete. I knew that birth, the beginning of life, was my calling and from then on, I was in regular contact with Donna via email and phone calls regarding questions I had about prenatal, labor, birth, and postpartum issues that would arise. She always has an answer for my questions and lovingly advises me through it all, even to this day. She is my mentor and dear friend. Because of her, I have experienced true love of midwifery.

My goal as a birth attendant is to bring pure strength back to moms and babies so families can be whole again. I truly believe with all my heart that when a mother goes through the miracle of birth the natural way and brings her baby into this world with her own raw strength, that she gathers from within, her ability to mother her babe the way the good Lord intended and her motherly affection is multiplied immensely. If all mothers would take the initiative to be healthier and deliver their babies naturally, the world would be a better place to raise our babies in.

I believe mothers are our society's strongest assets. Mothers are the heart of the family. With every beat of her heart she nurtures and strengthens her family. From conception to parenting their own, she teaches her children all of life's precious secrets. Body and soul feed on her knowledge. Husbands are blessed by her devoted love. Our world is defined by her ways. Let her ways be healthy and purposeful, full of love, laughter, and the calm reassurance that only a mother can give.

~5~
EXERCISES

Pelvic Rocks
Unborn babies are not mindless, masses of flesh. They are living beings that are eager to do things according to the laws of nature. All their instincts are intact, if we have not destroyed their natural foundation with unnatural things. When a baby has been taught how to find proper vertex (head down) position then, if baby moves, baby will usually be able to go back into position when directed.

The baby is floating in a bag of water, or more precisely amniotic fluid. The heaviest parts of the baby are the head and the spine. During the earlier months baby can swim around and move about. When baby gets older / bigger the living quarters are more cramped and baby tends to stay in one general place. Gravity can be used to position the baby if the proper exercises are done throughout the pregnancy. This cannot be done 'only' if there is a problem, but needs to be done on a regular basis, with the prime being 15 repetitions each morning and evening.

These exercises begin by getting down on ones hands and knees. The hands should be directly down from the shoulders and the knees should be wide enough apart to allow a full term baby's head to fit between the upper thighs. Mom's head is up. From this point, the back is dropped in order to let the belly hang toward the floor. This is going to allow the baby to slowly slide around and causes the spine to be facing the floor. Adjusting baby so the spine is not lying against mother's spine which relieves pressure off from mom's back and making life more comfortable for baby, too. This position should be held for about 20 seconds, or very slow count to 10. Remember, baby is floating in water and it takes baby longer to move than it does you. Be patient and let baby have the time needed.

Then change and drop the head down and tuck the bottom in tightly while arching the back up like a cat arching its back. (*as shown in the example*) This helps place baby's head down into the pelvis for a vertex position. Again hold for about 20 seconds and change back to the first position of head up and belly dropped. These exercises should be done each morning and evening for 15 repetitions (15 with the back arched up and 15 with the back dropped down) throughout the pregnancy, especially during the second and third trimesters. They can be done more frequently if mother feels it is needed for reasons such as the majority of the baby's movement is low, mother has a low backache, or baby appears to be laying transverse (sideways).

If there has been an accident where mother slips and falls on her bottom, it is not uncommon for baby to turn breech in order to protect his head. After a fall, it is recommended to do the exercises every hour or so throughout the day to put baby back where he belongs.

Squats
Squats are only done during the last couple of weeks before the estimated due date. The purpose of the squat is to place the baby's head against the cervix to assist in the dilation of the cervix and effacement.

Megan demonstrating
Pelvic Rocks

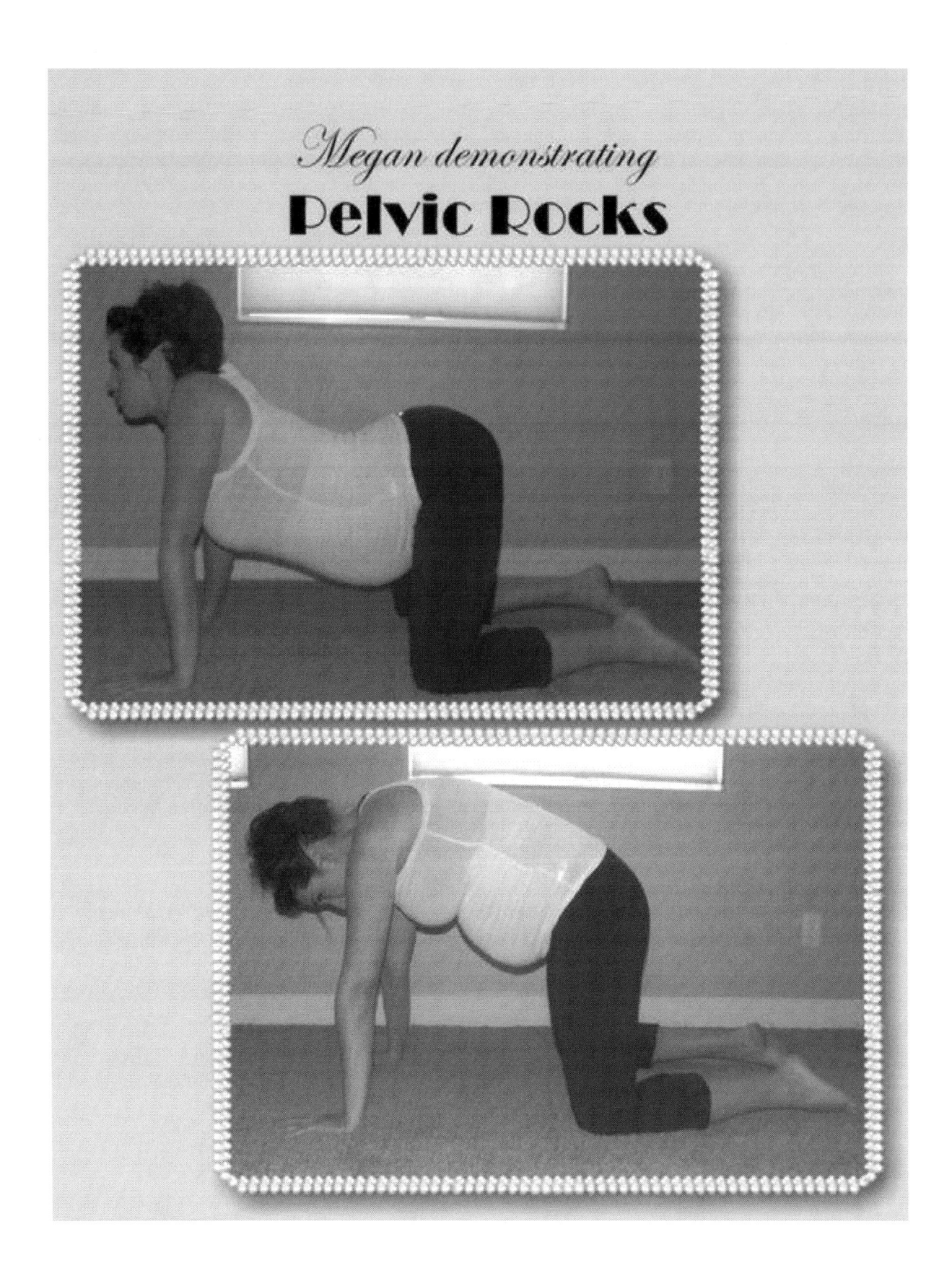

Megan demonstrating Squats

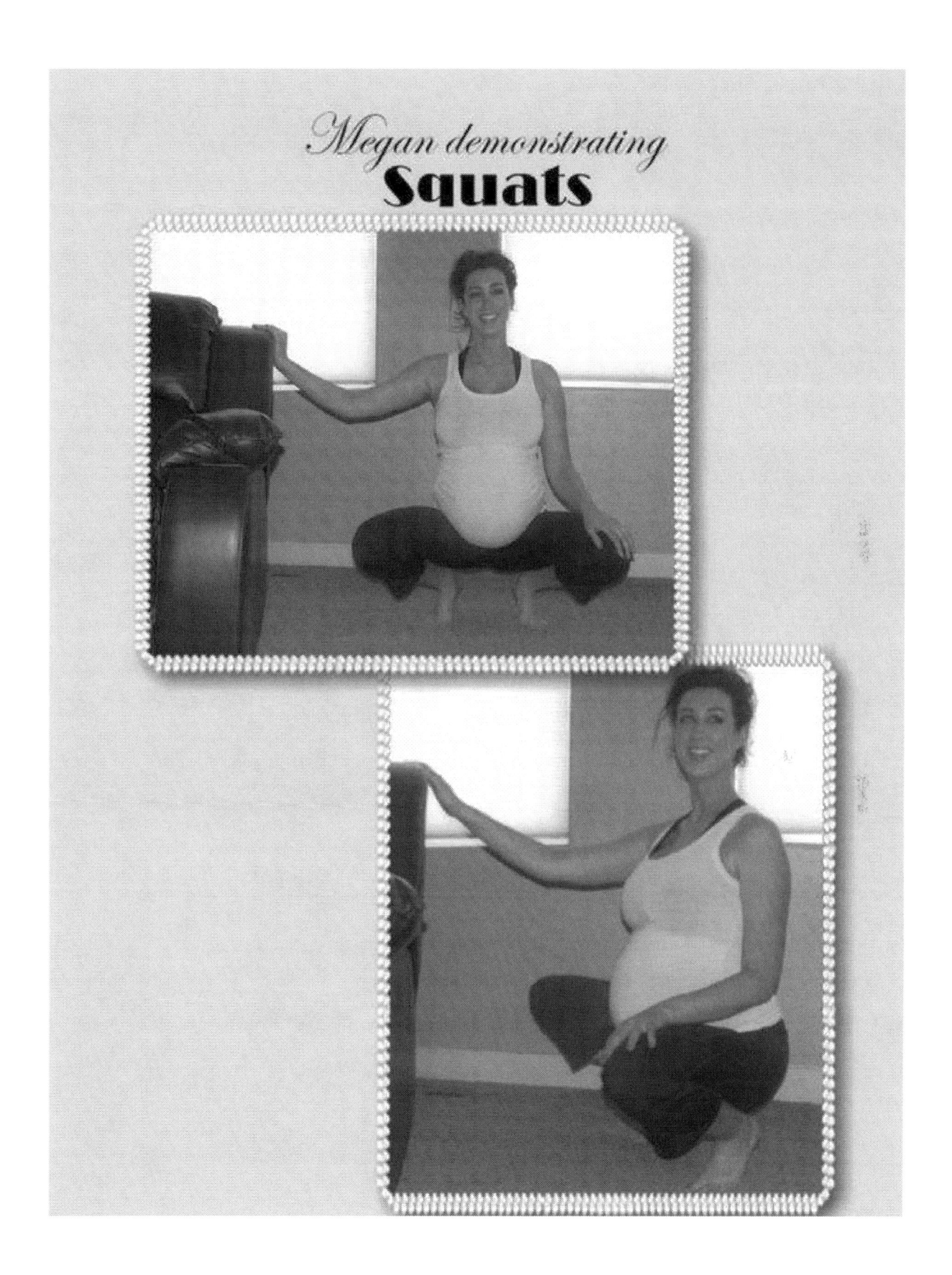

Megan demonstrating
Butterflies

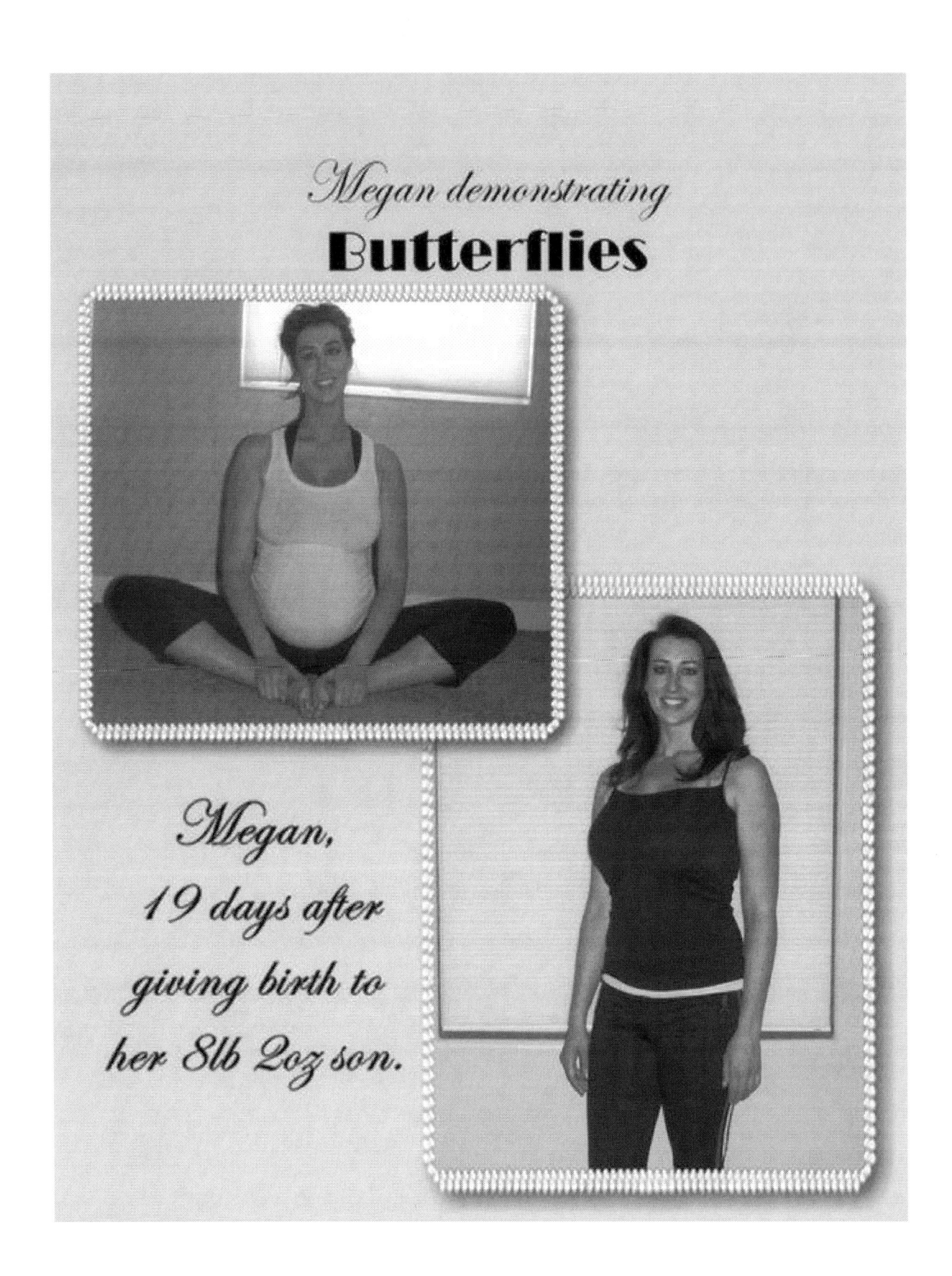

Megan, 19 days after giving birth to her 8lb 2oz son.

Many women have wonderful balance and coordination, even during pregnancy and do not need anything to hold on to. I recommend having a stable point to hold on to for safety reasons. The edge of a bed, a chair or coffee table, anything that won't tip and can assist in helping mom get to her feet if needed. Proper position for a squat is to go from a standing position, to straight down to almost sitting on the heels. The head is up and the back is straight. The knees are far enough apart that the baby's head has clear access to the cervix. The pictures show proper position from two angles.

Caution: Squats are not to be used if one already has a history of short labors or the healthcare provider is trying to hold baby inside longer.

Butterflies
Are used to stretch and strengthen the muscles next to the birth canal that, if pliable, allow the baby to descend through the birth canal a little faster causing a shorter 'push' time. These are done throughout the pregnancy, but the most important times are during the last two trimesters.

Begin by sitting on the floor with the back straight and the bottoms of the feet together. Pull the feet up as close to your bottom as you can. Using your elbows for gentle support, encourage the knees downward towards the floor. Do not push them to a point of pain, just stretch the muscles a little each day and within a few weeks the knees should come very close, if not completely, to the floor without effort.

Walking
Walking during pregnancy is an excellent form of exercise. It provides for increased circulation, lymphatic drainage and proper kidney and bowel function. Walking also strengthens the hips and legs as well as increasing oxygen assimilation and is good for every part of the body. I generally recommend walking about a mile a day beyond their normal work and family activities. I suggest walking at a good pace of two to three miles per hour for one mile, or more if desired.

Caution: Walking is not a good plan for anyone who is cramping or is having a potential miscarriage. It is always best to have someone else with you, just in case something happened such as a fall, or an accident. Later on in pregnancy it is wise to have someone with you to insure you do not go into labor while out on a walk and have difficulty getting home again.

It is not uncommon for walking to bring on mild contractions in the last trimester. Near labor, you may find that you contract while walking and then stop after you quit walking. Do not over-do the walking in an attempt to start labor as this usually leads to a woman starting her labor fatigued and that is never a good plan.

Walking stairs
During the last couple of weeks prior to the estimated due date, I will recommend walking stairs to assist in putting baby's head over the top of the cervix and using the baby's head to soften and thin the cervix to encourage a shorter labor time.

As always, it is best to have someone with you when walking stairs. Hold on to the guardrail and walk with the knees directly in front of you. Do not throw the knees out to the side as this prevents the effectiveness of the exercise.

Walking stairs works different muscles than walking on a flat surface. This is usually done directly after the pelvic rocks, which places the baby in the proper position. The stairs are intended to use the upper leg and thigh to rub the baby's head against the cervix and settle the baby down into birth position. Walking stairs for a maximum of 30 minutes is good, but do not go over 30 minutes as it will bring on sore muscles and fatigue. This should be performed two weeks prior to the EDD (estimated due date) until the birth.

Kegels
Kegels are the exercise that can be done while a woman is driving, sitting, watching TV, standing, going to the bathroom etc. The idea of the exercise is to strengthen and tone the muscles in the birth canal, urinary tract and pelvic floor.

Not intending to step on toes here, but I have a different attitude about this exercise than many. Kegels, also known as 'the elevator' exercise, are something that I hold off on until after baby is born. I object to our ladies using them during pregnancy. Although they are wonderful for intercourse, stopping urine flow and giving pelvic floor integrity. In my opinion, they are not good before childbirth. Nature itself does everything it can to soften and relax the birth canal the last few weeks before birth as to allow the passageway to be able to stretch for the baby to slide down and through. If the birth canal maintains firm muscle tone during this time it can equate into a much longer push time as well as increase the chances of a vaginal tear.

Within a few days after the birth, mother can start to do these exercises in order to restore vaginal muscle tone. The muscles being exercised are the ones in the vagina and the pelvic floor. If there is any doubt about the muscles they can be located in one of two ways. Slide a clean finger into the birth canal and then gently squeeze the muscles needed to tighten the vaginal muscles around the finger. Another way to assist in locating the muscle is when urinating. Squeeze the muscle to stop the urine flow and then release it. Both of these are using the same general muscles that are being used in the Kegel's exercises.

Kegels can be done by squeezing the muscles as tight as possible and then holding for about five seconds. As you tighten, take notice of how the muscles feel. Hold it for five seconds and then slowly relax the muscles. Wait about five seconds and then tighten again, repeating the same process about 10 times. When you tighten you will probably feel the tightening in the lower abdominal muscles also. Perform the exercise to see how many times it takes before the muscles begin to fatigue.

Once you have started these and understand the exercise, they can be increased to more repetitions and a longer duration. You may squeeze for 15 to 20 seconds before releasing. You will also be able to do more repetitions at a time. A nice time to perform the Kegels exercise is while traveling to the grocery store, folding clothes or doing computer work, etc. Performing Kegels three or four times a day is adequate after the birth until the next pregnancy. It is impossible to over-do this exercise after the birth. Plan on doing them for the rest of your life, and you will be glad you did.

~~~~~A Short Story~~~~~

A couple came to me and asked if I was capable of delivering a baby past a broken back. I asked them to explain and they told about how she had been in an accident where her lower back had been seriously damaged. This was years earlier, but the area still caused her grief on occasion. They explained that with the birth of their last child the doctor had put her in lithotomic position and had her push for hours before finally breaking the baby's collarbone as a means of helping the baby through the birth canal. I was sure I could birth a baby past the back injury and furthermore I was sure it could be done without damaging the baby. I agreed to take them as clients. They worked well as a team and did well at following instructions. When she went into labor her contractions would start and then stop, but finally she kicked into solid labor. As she did, the pain was mostly in her back and with each contraction she wanted lobelia extract (in an alcohol base), rubbed across her lower back and pressure points pressed. She did well and soon came the time for her to push. We moved into the bedroom where she could lie down, on her back, on the bed and I broke her water. During the next contraction she attempted to push and she said it hurt in her back. I had her attempt again for another couple of contractions and she said the pain was like it was in the hospital and it was an unnatural pain. By this time the baby was well started into the birth canal so a leak-proof pad was placed on the floor and I told her husband and the assistant, "On the count of three move her into a squat, right here. One, two, three." They lifted together to smoothly moved her into a squat. Within seconds, another contraction began and the baby's head was delivered. The cord was checked for and on the next contraction, seconds later, the rest of her baby was delivered. Instead of her push time being several hours, it was approximately 15 minutes with no damage to mother or child. Everyone was very happy.

NOTES_____

_____

_____

_____

_____

_____

_____

_____

_____

_____

~6~
HEIDI'S STORY

We have five children, four boys and one girl. From the beginning of our marriage, my husband and I wanted to find more natural ways to have our children. My mother had home births so that was something that we thought of looking into. We were kind of nervous because if you were at home and had any complications, then what were you supposed to do?

When we were pregnant with our first baby, we found someone in the Provo, Utah area to deliver our baby at home. It wasn't the experience that I was hoping for, the labor was very hard and long and I had some bleeding. This left me very apprehensive about having another baby.

We then moved to Jerome, Idaho where we met a woman, by the name of Donna Young. She changed our family's life, as far as the process of having our children was concerned. After I had my second baby, with Donna, I remember thinking, "Is that it? Is that all?" "Wow!" Donna helped me to control the bleeding and I was able to walk after I gave birth. Donna's technique is very helpful for expectant women; it makes the birthing process sacred, special, and something to look forward to. The attention was all on me having a baby and I never felt like I was "putting anyone out". It's your show, and your time. Having our children at home with Donna has been one of the most special and spiritual experiences we have had.

The diet and herbs help prepare your body for the birth. It is amazing that your body is able to work so well, with the things that God has put on the earth, to bring about the process of delivering a baby. Our baby came quickly because of the preparations prior to birth. Donna's technique prepares your body for an uncomplicated delivery and is designed to assist a woman's body as she prepares for childbirth.

On the day my daughter was born, I was up walking around and people were looking at me like, "What are you doing?" Women should have the opportunity to have children without being drugged or, incapable of going on with their lives. What an amazing and spiritual experience it can be, when you are in your home with your spouse and an educated birth attendant, who is conscientious and concerned about you. Donna has given my family and me something special that is sure to last in this life and through eternity. When our oldest son found out that Donna didn't help deliver him, he got quite upset because of the special connection he had witnessed with our babies.

Childbirth seems to be a topic that comes up frequently amongst mothers and I am continually amazed at their birth experiences. With my first baby I tore a lot, hemorrhaged, and I was not able to walk for a week. With the following babies (using Donna's technique) I never hemorrhaged and I was up walking the day of my delivery. If women could have this knowledge of how to take care of themselves during pregnancy, so many complications could be avoided. I am continually amazed with our body's ability, to do what they were intended to do, when we learn to take care of them. It is not supposed to be complicated.

I have been thinking lately about my daughter's future and it makes me nervous about how standardized birth has become. Most care providers don't seem to have a complete understanding of how the body works and either do women. This causes unnecessary complications to arise. If we could have understanding on both ends, we would have many more rewarding deliveries. This book will be my gift to my daughter and daughters-in-law in hopes that they will be able to have positive birth experiences.

Powerfully Pregnant

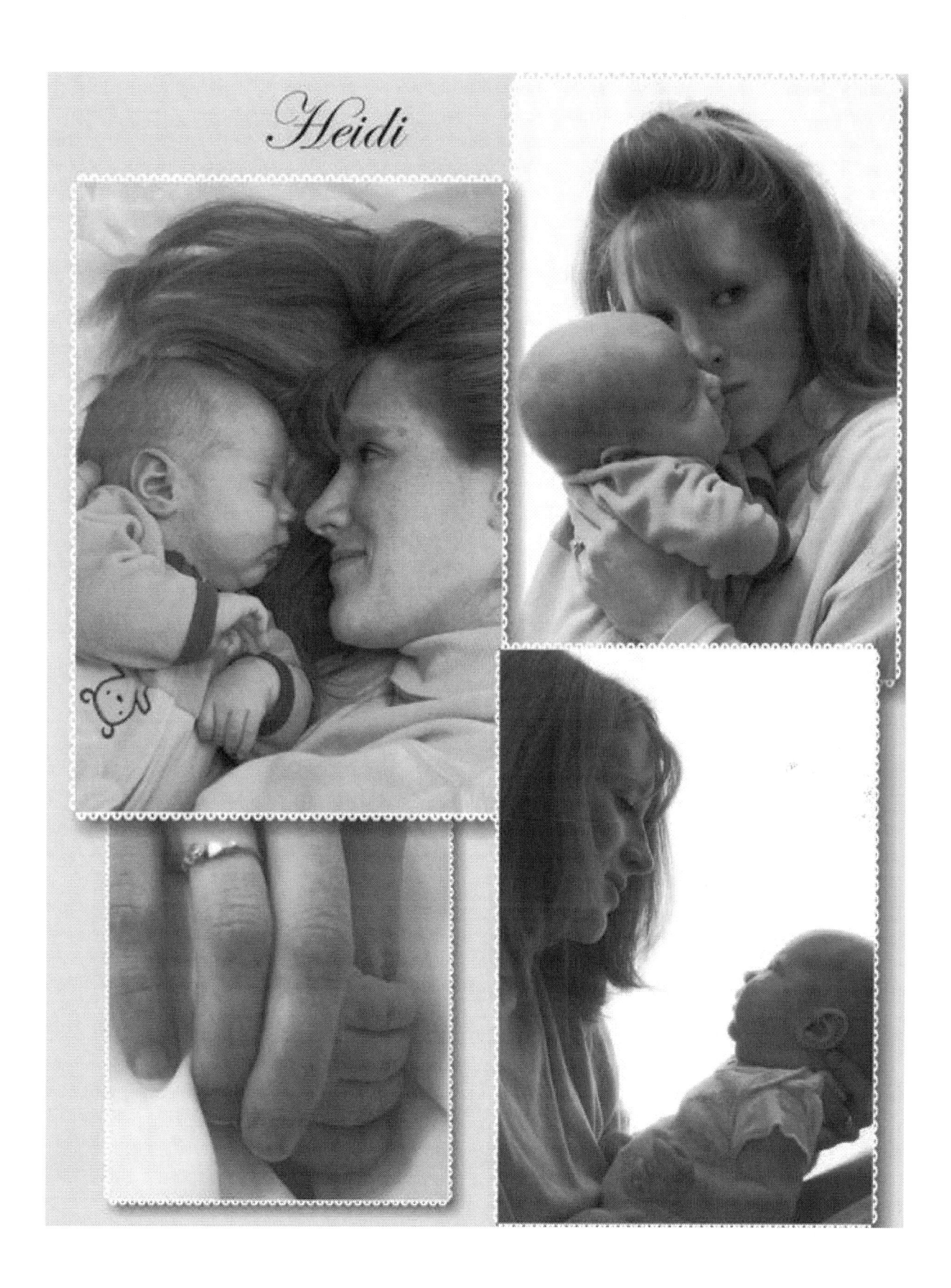

Heidi

Women were made to have babies, God gave us this ability and we are the ones that have complicated the whole process. If we were to purify and simplify the birthing process, it would eliminate many unnecessary challenges. The birthing process is not supposed to be hard. Women should be able to walk away without all of the 'baggage'. Tearing, complications from drugs, and c-sections take away from the beautiful, sacred and rewarding experience of birth, making it harder for women to ever want another baby.

If there was any advise that I could give to other women it would be, *"Listen to your body. Take those things into it that will help prepare your body for labor. It is the best thing you can do for you and your baby. You are in control."*

~7~
PRENATAL CARE

Prenatal exams are the time when most complications are found during pregnancy. If found, and recognized during this time, they have less chance to build into a major problem. Problems should be resolved as soon as they are found in order to limit complications during the birth.

If there is a problem, then we discuss the problem, the cause and the solution. It takes knowledge to recognize the problems and it takes discipline to bring resolution. This section is meant to increase your knowledge so that you may exercise the discipline to resolve the majority of problems that may arise during pregnancy. It takes a little longer to do things this way, but the results are well worth it. Again, it is all personal responsibility.

These are the things I evaluate at every prenatal exam:

Urine Test

First a urine sample is taken. The sample is taken into a clean, disposable container like a clean paper cup (¼ to ½ cup of urine is plenty).

I use a 10 parameter urinalysis strip. There are several companies that make them, and can be picked up either online or from most pharmacies. The idea is to make sure they have all ten spots to test each of the areas. Each container has 100 strips (they also have an expiration date) so you will have extras after the pregnancy so use them freely, especially if you are trying to keep an eye on any issues that arise. It is certainly a non-invasive way to check for things.

Once the urine is in the cup. I take one of the test strips out of the container, immediately replacing the lid, and dip the strip into the urine. It does not need to soak just lay it along the side of the cup and tip the cup to cover each spot on the strip then remove the strip and dry off the back of the strip, with a piece of toilet paper, to remove excess urine and prevent any of the urine from mixing the chemicals in the different parameters. I DO NOT TOUCH THE FRONT OF THE STRIP as this can alter the chemicals. Wait 30-60 seconds before reading the strip. Then compare the color of the parameters to the chart on the side of the container. The strip is going to check for Blood, Urobilinogen, Bilirubin, Protein, Nitrites, Ketones, Glucose, Specific Gravity, pH and Leukocytes. Following are brief explanations of what these readings mean and basic suggestions.

Blood: The parameter for blood is generally yellow and if the parameter turns green then this shows there is blood in the urine. The darker the shade of green, the higher the concentration of blood there is in the urine. The amount of blood tells us different things. Throughout most of the pregnancy there should be no signs of blood. Trace amounts (pale green) generally show there has been a disturbance of the cervix. Lovemaking, athletics such as horse riding, volleyball, or moderate lifting etc. If this is accounted for then there is not a problem, as long as it is never increased. If there has been no activity that would disturb the cervix, then it needs to be watched to insure there are no pending problems. Trace amounts of blood can be a sign of dilation. This is expected during the final days before delivery, but if it happens earlier in the pregnancy then it is not good and appropriate measures should be taken.

Another cause for blood showing up in the urine would be a UTI (urinary tract infection). If there is an infection then there will generally be a show of protein and leukocytes along with the blood. Any show of blood other than a lighter color on the strip, without reason, should result in light activity. If a darker color shows up on the strip then one should be on bed rest. Anything that is 'visible-to the naked eye' in the cup is an absolute reason for bed rest until the problem can be resolved. A healthy pregnancy does not have breakthrough bleeding. Any visible sign of blood during pregnancy is unacceptable. (*See Trouble Shooting Miscarriages section for more information*)

Possible solution: As long as there is no high blood pressure or excess iron, then a ferrous sulfate found in most pharmacies, can be taken one tablet per day to restore the iron levels, prevent anemia and lessen the chances of bleeding.

Ferrum Phos. 6X (Cell salt #4) found where supplements are sold can be taken to lessen blood loss. When the Ferrum Phos is taken I expect to see a noticeable change in a short amount of time, usually about 15 minutes or less and doses are repeated anytime there is any increase of show. If blood shows up in the urine a dose of Ferrum Phos is taken three times a day until all show is absent from the urine test.

Increasing the amounts of spinach and beets in the diet is also a good plan.

Urobilinogin and Bilirubin are primary compounds produced by the liver. Elevations on either of these parameters show there is a problem somewhere in the liver. The two tend to balance each other and if there is an over production then the liver is working too hard. The Bilirubin is a yellow / orange color that gives the yellow tinge to urine, to bruises, and the yellow discoloration in jaundice. Urobilinogin is colorless in the liver but turns brown when oxidized in the intestine giving the stool its characteristic brown color. If Urobilinogin and Bilirubin show up in a urine test, this would be a red flag for issues such as hepatitis or other liver ailments, but these parameters will generally show up with leukocytes and sometimes nitrites if that were the case. Most generally when either of these show up in the urine test it is an enzyme imbalance.

Possible Solution: Stop eating the foods that are hard on the liver, such as fatty foods, carbonation, sugars, potatoes, corn, and heat producing foods. Take a look at your water source and make sure your water is free of chemicals, parasites and toxins.

If needed, pick up a water purification system. There are some really good ones out on the market. Read up on available brands to see which best fits your needs and are within your price range.

Drink several tall glasses of apple juice every day for a few days. Historically, apple juice has been used to assist in liver cleanses / flushes. (This is not a possibility for anyone who has high blood sugar issues.)

I recommend my ladies take two to three ginger root capsules (or ½ to ¾ tsp. bulk ginger) before each meal to help with liver function. A broad based food enzyme, which helps digest fats, proteins, carbohydrates, sugars and dairy would work in place of the ginger.

If these measures do not show resolution then further examination by a health care professional is probably in order. You can get a second opinion from an honest health care provider who is willing to support your decisions.

Protein in the urine is showing that the kidneys are not filtering properly. This will show up in the case of a urinary tract infection, poor protein assimilation, and in conditions of weakened kidneys.

Possible Solution: Increase the amount of water to dilute the concentration of solid parts per million in the urine. Higher concentrations tend to make the kidneys work harder.

I generally suggest the kidneys be nutritionally supported with an herbal combination that has dandelion, uva ursi, marshmallow, parsley, juniper and chamomile. Tea or capsule is fine. Suggested dose is two capsules three times per day (or one cup two to three times per day of the tea).

Then, if protein is not being broken down and assimilated, I suggest mixing unsweetened beef gelatin with warm liquid and drinking it with each meal. This helps provide protein in a form that is easily assimilated by the body without adding pressure to the kidneys.

Nitrites indicate possible bacteria in the urine. This shows when there are bacterial infection(s) anywhere in the body.
Possible solution: I question my ladies about other possible signs of infection such as discharges, inflammations, swellings, chills, fevers etc. If infection is surfacing in a specific area then that area can be watched for signs of change for either improvement or worsening. Such as, if there is a sinus infection, does it improve or worsen with treatment? This tells us if we are getting results without a urine test. We call this 'Listening to our body'.

Stop all sugar, carbonation and milk. Drink extra water or herbal teas to thin the concentration of infection for easier transport out of the body.

Every time nitrites show up in the urine I suggest a natural supplement that has been historically used for bacterial infections. Two capsules of golden seal root (not intended for long term use or for ladies with low blood sugar-hypoglycemia) taken three times per day for a couple of weeks and/or two droppers full of colloidal silver 1100ppm taken three times a day for a couple of weeks. Occasionally these will both need to be taken together.

Immune support is also suggested while there are signs of infections, with supplements such as IP-6, garlic, and echinacea at the recommended amounts.

A lightening on the parameter should be seen in just a day or two. If there are any increasing symptoms such as fever, chills or pain then contacting a health care professional is in order. If there is not a health care provider available then increasing amounts to the recommended dose every waking hour for one to two days and then cutting back as necessary should prevent further infection. Nitrites need to be brought into order in a short time to prevent miscarriage or further bacterial damage. With any of my ladies who show nitrites, I do a recheck in 24-48 hours to check for signs of improvement, if they are not making expected progress then I suggest they seek medical attention.

Ketones result from either diabetic ketosis or else caloric deprivation. This happens with weight loss if there are not adequate amounts of nutrition going into the body. Proper nutrition will allow the body to regulate weight without ketosis. Conditions such as starvation (not taking in nutrition), morning sickness (vomiting ingested foods) etc. will cause the muscle to break down to keep the organs going. If there are ketones showing, there is improper weight loss happening.
Possible solution: Stop milk, sugar and carbonation. Increase the amount of easily assimilated protein such as unsweetened beef gelatin in warm vegetable, beef or chicken broth. Eat more meals of smaller portions. Protein also assists in balancing the blood sugar. If the cause is elevated glucose, the glucose parameter on the strip will also show then follow instructions for gestational diabetes are given, listed in the Second Trimester chapter. Signs of improvement should be seen within one week as well as improvement in the ketone parameter, if instructions are being followed.

Glucose: is a sign that too much sugar is in the system. This is generally caused from eating improper carbohydrates or else too many carbohydrates.
Possible Solution: Stop eating sugar, breads, potatoes and corn. Increase the amount of protein in the diet.

If the amount of glucose is more than 'slightly' elevated then golden seal root at doses of 2 capsules 3 times a day is usually suggested along with diet for the next two weeks. By then the body should have increased the insulin production to a normal level. Again, if the levels are not brought into line within a couple of weeks then she may need to see a health care professional.

Specific Gravity: shows how many parts, per million solid sediments, there are in the urine. In other words, how concentrated (dense) the urine is. If elevated, this shows lack of water consumption. This shows the fluid intake is not keeping up with the body's needs.
Possible solution: Drink more water to thin the urine and other body fluids. Note: only water and herbal teas are considered proper fluids for this purpose. Carbonation, juices and sugared drinks add to the problem.

pH: Checks for the balance between acidity and alkaline in the body. The proper pH balance for humans should be slightly acidic at five and a half to six and a half. (5.5 to 6.5) If the body is alkaline then it cannot break down the nutrients as nature intended. Water is neutral at a pH of seven. If the body is over acidic, which is common in our society, then there can be heartburn, acid indigestion and, in the long run, a colicky baby. It can also lead to things like arthritis and gout.
Possible solution: If the urine shows anything over a pH of seven then the "No high acid foods" rule can be broken. I generally recommend a glass of pineapple, orange or grapefruit juice a couple of times per week. This is the only exception to the rule.

If the ph is below 5.5 then the body is too acidic and can cause heartburn, acid reflux or arthritic symptoms. Stop putting high acid food and drinks into the body and increase the amount of calcium.

Leukocytes: are a sign that white blood cells have given their lives to infection. This can be any kind of infection (bacterial, viral, yeast). This can be anything from a cold to a urinary tract infection. All infections eventually make their way to the urinary tract in order get out of the body.
Possible solution: Stop the foods that add to infection or lower the immune system such as milk, sugar, carbonation and pork. Drink plenty of water.

I suggest taking an infection-fighting supplement such as yarrow (not for anyone with high blood pressure) or garlic for viral, goldenseal root or colloidal silver for bacterial, or caprylic acid or grapefruit seed extract for yeast infections. Starting with the dosing recommendation on the bottle and then increasing if needed. Urine tests every 24 hours can show whether or not progress is being made. I suggest staying with any type of infection-fighting supplement for seven days past any symptoms, before stopping.

I also suggest N-Acetyl Cysteine to support the production of new, healthy white blood cells at recommended amounts (on the bottle) for the next 3-4 weeks after leukocytes clear in the urine.

If a urine test shows protein, leukocytes and nitrites there is probably a urinary tract infection (UTI) going on. This needs to be recognized and dealt with immediately.

Weight
The weight is taken at each appointment using the same set of scales each time. Scales vary, so to

track the weight we have to have a base point. I buy the same brand of scales when they need to be replaced as to keep accuracy.

There has been controversy, lately on how much weight a woman should gain during pregnancy and the excessive weight gain during pregnancy has been thought to cause problems with obesity in children. I feel a healthy pregnancy, for an average sized woman, should have enough weight gain to cover baby, placenta and water. Anything else I consider to be "extra" weight that a mother-to-be does not need to have. If a woman is under weight or not yet matured then we expect the weight to come up and regulate. An overweight woman can safely lose weight while growing a healthy, seven (plus) pound baby if she is eating a balanced and healthy diet. I do not like to see underweight women lose weight or show ketones in their urine. This shows they are not getting their nutritional needs met.

Young ladies who are not fully developed prior to getting pregnant will mature during pregnancy. The body will develop and finish filling out and this type of weight gain is acceptable and even appreciated.

During the first five months of pregnancy, I expect to see very little weight gain because the fetus weighs less than a pound until about the 24th week and the placenta and amniotic fluid also total less than a pound. If the mother-to-be has put on 15 pounds then I know that the other 13 pounds is extra weight. Women, who gain extra weight during their pregnancy, tend to suffer more from post partum depression because the weight left to lose requires work or has to be lived with. Neither is the preferred outcome. On the other hand, women who look good and feel good after the birth are far less prone to suffer from Post Partum Depression.

During the last month of pregnancy the baby gains about a half a pound per week, so it is expected that there will more gain during this time, without a change in diet.

Another cause of weight gain is pre-eclampsia also called toxemia. This is where the liver and kidneys are not able to accommodate the toxin levels in the body and there is excessive weight gain, generally accompanied with an elevation in blood pressure. I feel that pre-eclampsia is a problem that can be avoided if a woman will start exercising and will go the extra mile to avoid the foods that can cause the problem such as carbonation, flour products and sugars.

Possible solutions for being underweight: For underweight ladies or weight loss with ketones in the urine. Try to find the solution to morning sickness (*found in the First Trimester section*), do not skip any meals, and increase the amount of protein being eaten. Unsweetened beef gelatin is easily assimilated and is easy on the stomach. Take ginger or food enzymes to help aid the body in digesting foods for proper liver function.

Possible solutions for excess weight gain: Stop the breads (all flour products), sugar, carbonation, potatoes and corn. Eating, even healthy meals, too close to going to bed will cause weight gain. Eat the last meal at least three hours prior to bedtime.

Remember to eat for nutrition not for "cravings".

Take time to walk at least a mile per day to assist the lymphatic system, kidneys and bowels to perform as intended by nature.

Carbonation is a primary reason for the filtering system (liver, kidneys and spleen) to shut down causing weight gain and high blood pressure. All carbonated beverages need to be stopped. Even sparkling mineral water is hard on the body and can result in weight gain and elevated blood pressure.

Blood pressure

Blood pressure tells the amount of fluid volume in the body. The top number (systolic) tells the amount of pressure against the vessel wall when the heart is beating. The bottom number (diastolic) tells the amount of pressure against the vessel wall when the heart is in a resting state. If the top number is high it shows that there is a heavy pressure against the blood vessel(s) when the heart beats. If the bottom number is too high then it shows there is excess pressure against the blood vessel(s) wall when the heart is resting between beats. Meaning the heart and blood vessels never get a break from the pressure.

A healthy heart and circulatory system will generally reflect a blood pressure of about 115-120 / 65-70, which tells us that the heart has an adequate amount of blood moving through the system with a minimal amount of pressure to the heart, brain, veins and/or arteries.

High blood pressure: There may be no symptoms of high blood pressure (this is why it is known as the "silent killer"), but there can be signs such as headaches, pounding in the chest, or the ability to visibly see the vein on the neck moving with each heartbeat. Frustration, irritability and nervousness can also accompany higher blood pressure.

If the blood pressure is too high during pregnancy, than this puts mother at risk for a heart attack or stroke during labor because of the already stressed system being under even more pressure with the efforts of labor. The blood pressure rises by a small amount, routinely, when a person is in pain or under stress due to the added adrenaline production. It is reckless to attempt labor in a woman with high blood pressure, anything with a top reading (systolic) over 150 or a bottom reading (diastolic) over 90. The blood pressure needs to be brought under control or the birth needs to take place in a controlled environment. High blood pressure is a good reason to transport during a home birth. (*For specific information on suggestions for treating high blood pressure, see Blood Pressure in the Second Trimester chapter*)

Low blood pressure: Equally concerning, as high blood pressure is low blood pressure. If the top number (systolic) falls below 100 or the bottom number (diastolic) falls below 50 it signifies there is not enough blood volume in the body to keep adequate blood flow. Symptoms of low blood pressure are generally fatigue, dizziness, visual disturbances, and/or weakness. I have also noticed that ladies who have low blood pressure are more prone, than those women who have a normal blood pressure reading, to hemorrhage during and after the birth of their baby. (*For information on suggestions to treat low blood pressure see fatigue / dizziness in the First Trimester chapter*)

Pulse

A pulse should be taken in a resting state, either sitting or lying down, with as little noise as possible. A pulse should be taken for a minimum of 15 seconds, but I prefer to take the pulse for 30 seconds to a minute. The average pulse rate for athletes is about 58-62 per minute. The average pulse rate for an expectant mother should be 64-72, with athletic mothers being slightly lower. A pulse is taken by placing two fingers (not your thumb) over an artery and counting how many times it pulses in one minute. You can count the number of beats in 15 seconds and then multiply this number by four, or count the number of beats in 30 seconds and multiply by two, to get a full minute count.

If the heart is beating too fast it generally shows either stress, lack of calcium being assimilated, or low blood pressure. We locate the cause and then resolve the problem.

If the beat is irregular, the heart may be in need of more nutrients and generally is due to a lack of calcium or overall minerals. She may need electrolytes or the thyroid is in need of more attention. We look for other symptoms to find the exact cause then treat accordingly.

I have come to the conclusion that, "If the heart beats too fast it is under stress and needs a calmative such as calcium (not from a rock base). If the heart beats to slow it needs nutritional support such as hawthorn berries."

Edema or Swelling
I will look at the hands and feet to see if there is any swelling in the fingers, toes or ankles (a ring or impression around her leg where the sock was). Swelling is a sign that the kidneys are not doing their job to run excess fluid off the system. If the excess fluid is left on the system it will cause bigger problems than just puffy extremities, it leads to water backup throughout the system resulting in conditions such as high blood pressure and pre-eclampsia. (*For information on suggestions to treat edema see edema/ water retention in the Second Trimester section.*)

Uterine Fundal Measurement
To measure the growth of the baby, the uterus is measured, in centimeters, by measuring from the top of the pubic bone to the top of the uterus (fundus). This can be difficult to find for an inexperienced person during the first 12 weeks of pregnancy. After that it should be fairly well defined and easy to locate as the uterus firms up and the outline is more visible. It is best to measure right after a woman has done her pelvic rock exercises, so that the baby is always in the same position when being measured.

As a rule, by about 16 weeks the top of the fundus is at about 16 centimeters (about to the naval on the average sized woman) and will gain a centimeter per week until the last couple of weeks. During the 24th week of pregnancy the uterus should measure 23-25 centimeters.

By about the 37th week of pregnancy, the fundal height will measure a little larger as the baby is growing and gaining weight more rapidly. The uterus will grow to about 40 centimeters by about the 39th week and then the measurement will drop back down by about three to four centimeters when a woman's body begins to prepare for labor. This drop is caused from a woman's hips relaxing outward to allow the baby to settle down into the pelvis. From the time of the drop until birth it is generally seven to ten days, but can be as soon as a few hours.

Smaller built women will measure a few weeks smaller during pregnancy and may never have a fundal height over 36 centimeters which is fine as long as she is maintaining a healthy lifestyle without drugs, tobacco, alcohol, etc., and is eating a healthy diet.

If the measurement of the uterus is growing rapidly, this can be a sign of a multiple pregnancy or can be a sign of too much amniotic fluid. In the event of an increased fundal measurement a woman should have things checked out by ultra sound. The excess amniotic fluid is very doubtful if she is eating properly, exercising, and the kidneys are functioning properly. If the uterus were growing at a rate of two centimeters per week instead of one, then it would be a good idea to have things checked to find out the cause. Even in a woman that is obese, there should not be a doubling of fundal height. The fundal height is a way to tell what is happening inside the uterus.

If a woman is measuring normal and then stops growing, it can mean the baby has changed positions (went from laying up and down to side to side). If she does her exercises and then the measurement comes up it is due to the change of position of the baby.

If the measurement does not come up, then locating the fetal heart tone would be the next thing to check. If the fetal heat tone is there and audible then we know baby is alive, but is probably not getting adequate nutrition. If there is no change in measurement and no audible fetal heart tone then there is a high possibility of a deceased baby. This would generally coincide with feeling no movement and requires immediate medical attention.

Fetal Heart Tone and Cord Sounds
When checking for the baby's heartbeat I use a Doppler. A Doppler runs on sound waves and is safe to use as long as it is not over used. A Doppler is great at picking up the heart and cord sounds as well as potential irregularities.

The cord sounds are easier to find as the cord grows longer and floats around in the amniotic sac. The cord has no valves, and so there is just the sound of the blood pulsating through the cord. When listening to the cord it has a sound that is similar to, without using the throat and only using the mouth to say, "wow-wow-wow-wow". The cord sound should beat at the same pace as the heartbeat. The tone of the cord should be regular and smooth in rhythm.

The sound of the heartbeat is located between the baby's shoulder blades and has the valves in the heart that open and close with each beat, giving a different sound that is more like, "plop-plop, plop-plop," which is distinctively different. I listen for a regular, consistent rhythm, and the number of beats per minute with the average being around 140. There should be a clear "snap" heard if the valve is opening and closing correctly. If a "whooshing" sound is heard, without the clear action of the valve, then this shows a potential heart problem in the baby and needs to be looked into further.

While listening for the fetal heart tone we divide the belly into quarters, figuratively, with the naval as the center point.

The cord goes from the placenta to the naval of the baby and it moves as the child moves. The heart can change depending on the position of the baby and as long as the heartbeat is located in the lower half of the belly then the baby is head down. If the heartbeat is found in the upper half of the belly then we know the baby is breech, meaning lying with the head up and the bottom down, which makes for a difficult birth and some states mandate breeches be c-sectioned. (*to learn more about a breech baby read the Third Trimester section and the section on pregnancy exercises.*) I stress strongly that laws be followed, if you don't like the laws in your state then either help get the laws changed through your representatives or else move to another state where you do like the laws. If you have not been successful at turning baby to the proper, head down/ vertex, position before the birth then a birth attendant who is experienced in delivering breeches needs to be involved or arrangements for a c-section need to be made, depending on the laws in that state.

Shortly before the birth, I generally check for the sound of the cord close to the pubic bone to see if there is a cord around the neck. If the sound of the cord is found all the way across the lower abdomen then preparations need to be made during the birth to accommodate for a cord wrapped around the neck. If the sound of the cord is audible on only one side, or the other, then we know it is around one shoulder or hanging low, which tells us to use extra caution when the water breaks and check for a prolapsed cord. Being watchful during prenatal care helps to avoid surprise complications during labor and delivery.

Answer all questions Women have questions that need answers and the answers to those questions should come from the care provider. I am on call for our ladies 24/7 for emergencies but the bulk of the questions or concerns are resolved during prenatal exams.

NOTES_____

~8~
LYNDSY'S STORY

In September of 2009, my husband and I found out that we were expecting our first baby. We were so thrilled to become parents. Both sides of the family were so supportive and happy to become grandparents.

I started going to an OB/GYN for the first few months of my pregnancy, but then as the third month went by we decided that we were not happy with our experience. We started looking for a midwife that lived near us and that is when we found Donna. On the initial visit with Donna, I learned more in 30 minutes than I had in the last three months and I loved the fact that she had answers and solutions to problems. She never rushed in and out of our home, she was always so kind, and made sure that my husband, baby, and I were doing well.

Donna told me that I had to follow her program, if she was going to do the birth and it was hard at first, but after we changed our eating habits I felt so much better. When I started eating healthy the morning sickness and heartburn went away, I had so much energy, I felt healthy, and at 20 weeks along I was able to go lion hunting with my husband. I loved being pregnant.

As the months passed by, I started experiencing some depression. I called Donna and she suggested a couple different herbs and I started feeling better again. I loved the fact that she was able to help me by using natural remedies.

The last few weeks of my pregnancy seemed to drag on and I was so ready to hold our baby. Three days after my due date at 3:00 AM I started having contractions. I decided to call Donna and she quickly came over to see how my labor was progressing and found that I was dilated four centimeters. Donna had me walking up and down the stairs and as I paced around the house things started getting more intense. Donna then broke my water and it really helped my labor to progress. I had a lot of family there waiting for the arrival of the baby and I finally decided that this was why my labor wasn't progressing and had to send everyone away. I walked up and down our street for a little while then decided to go take a bath at my mom's house next door. When I got out of the bath I was dilated to eight centimeters.

I went back to my house and by then was ready to start pushing. During one of my pushes, a gush of fluid gushed out and splashed Donna right in the face, everyone started laughing and I said to her," I want to laugh so bad right now but I'm just in too much pain. I will laugh later." A few pushes on the birth stool and my little seven pound four ounce boy finally made his arrival. Donna was so calm the entire time and knew exactly what to do.

When I first became pregnant I weighed 115 pounds and my weight just before I had the baby was 130 pounds. Within six weeks of the birth of my baby I was back down to my pre-pregnancy weight.

I was so happy that we decided to have a home birth. I never had to adjust the baby into a new environment and I loved that I was home, where I was comfortable.

Lyndsy at 40 Weeks

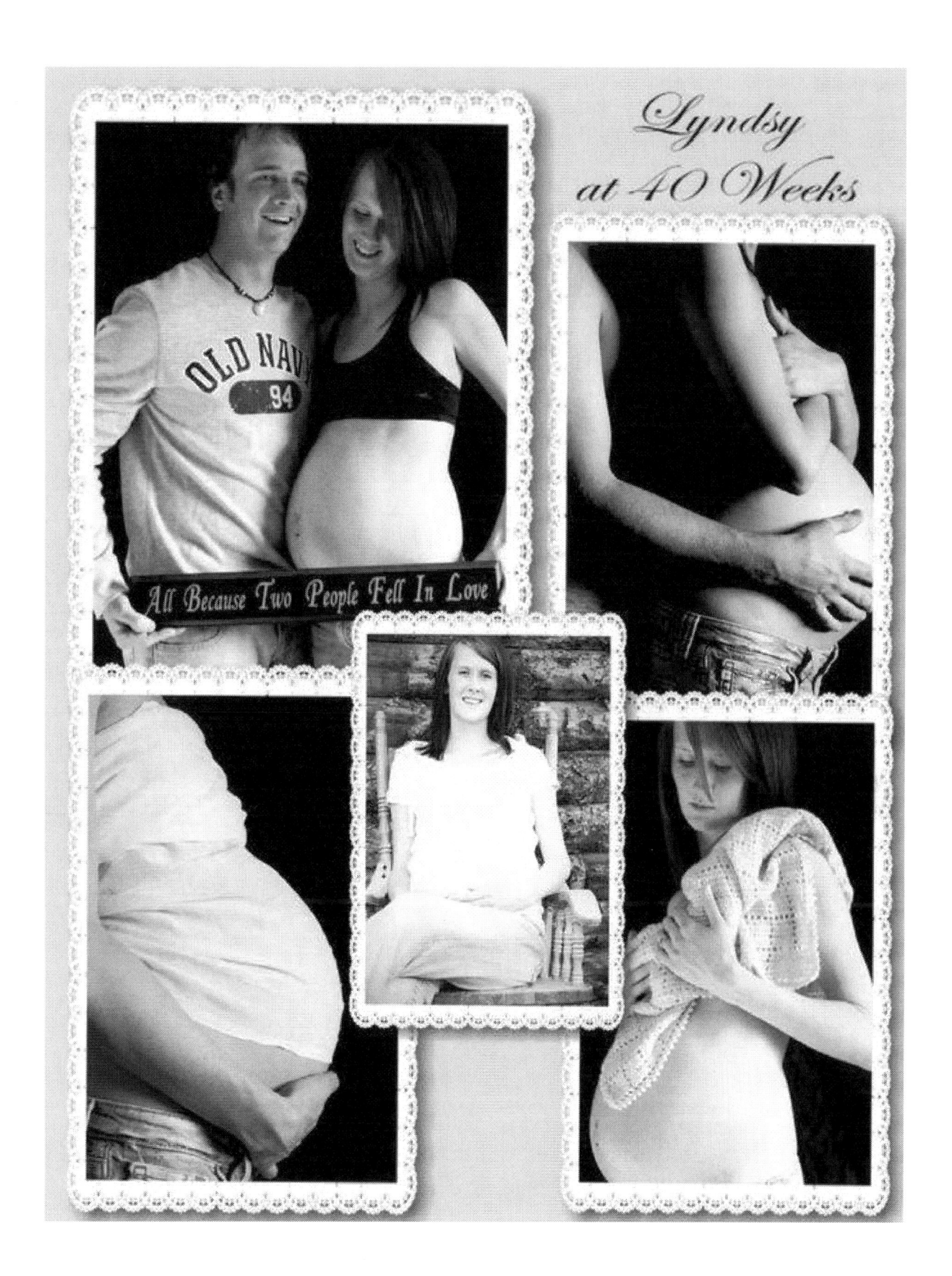

~9~
MISCARRIAGES

Emotions

I once received a call from a married man with eight children. His wife was pregnant with their ninth child and started to miscarry. His wife was losing large amounts of blood and the nearest hospital was over 75 miles away. He knew that there was not enough time to take his wife to the hospital without losing her. He asked me over the phone what could be done to help his wife. I walked them through the different herbs and homeopaths to help control the bleeding. After working with her for a while he was finally able to get the bleeding stopped. His wife was very weak, but would recover.

A couple of weeks after their loss, I received a phone call from the wife telling me that she was upset at her husband for being selfish and that he did not seem to understand how much emotional pain she had over the loss of her child. I then told her that I understood her loss, the pain that she was feeling and agreed that there is nothing that can ever replace the loss of a child. I then began to explain to her, "You are not the only one that lost a child, your husband did too. Your husband almost lost you too and can you imagine the pain he has endured? Have you stopped to think of what he has gone through? Have you stopped to thank him for saving your life? Please try to understand where he is coming from and put your arms around him and tell him that you are sorry and that you love him. I know that he will do his part, he is a good man." She told me she had been so busy feeling her own loss that she had not thought of his and she was going to love her husband unconditionally and with those words she hung up the phone.

A week or so later I received a letter that she had written:
"I just wanted to thank you for giving me my life back. If it wasn't for your knowledge and willingness to help I would not be here today. I am so grateful for life. Much more than I was 2 ½ - 3 weeks ago.

I also wanted you to know that I appreciate the chastisement that you gave me on the phone. I really did need to hear those things. I was so worried about (him) needing to change that I did not look where I needed to look-in the mirror! I had to realize that I am the only one who can change me.... We are getting along better than we ever have. We are taking time for each other and expressing our love and appreciation from the heart for each other. It's so great! I don't want to lose this feeling.

I just wanted you to know how dear you are to me and I thank the Lord for your friendship and love. May God Bless you in this great service that you are giving to so many women at one of the most precious times of their lives--Childbearing--You are an angel. I love you Donna!

P.S. I will keep in touch!"

The unexpected loss of a wanted pregnancy can be one of the greatest strains on a relationship. Most of the time the woman blames herself because she feels that she didn't do a good enough job at taking care of the baby. She starts to think that if she could have done something different or something better then the baby would still be alive. The woman may feel like she let her husband down and it may be hard for a woman to put into words the many emotions and thoughts that are running through her head. "Is something wrong with my body? Why can't my body carry a baby? Am I inept inside? Was it something I did? Why did I lose this baby? If I don't know what I did wrong, how can I prevent this from happening again? I don't feel worthy of my husband's love. I cannot go through losing another child. I know, he knows, it was my fault. Then a woman withdraws and doesn't communicate.

The husband/father has lost a baby that he wanted so much and now his wife won't talk to him and he begins to wonder, "Is she blaming me?" "Why won't she talk to me?" "Why won't she let me hold her?" "Why is she shutting me completely out?" "Why won't she even look directly at me?" "Doesn't she understand, that she is not the only one hurting here?" He needs to be held and needs her to talk; after all, he lost a baby too. A husband may even begin to wonder, "Why am I losing everything that means so much to me?" "Why?" Then he desperately tries to search for things he did wrong to make his wife turn away from him, during a time of such loss, and he cannot find an answer.

It is a tough situation. It is hard on both and neither knows how to talk to the other. The pain seems too great and a couple may soon feel it is easier to express anger than it is to feel pain and guilt. Pain and guilt are internalized and, eventually, make the chest feel like it is going to explode. At that point there is physical discomfort that goes along with the over powering sorrow. Anger is externalized, it is vented, but it allows the physical discomfort to be released, resulting in a better ability to cope. When there is an out-lashing of anger, separation usually follows and if something does not change, before this point, it can destroy the relationship. Anger can drive a wedge between them that may never heal back.

To the Husband/Father: To avoid letting the situation turn to anger, the first step could come from the husband. From several feet away, without touching her, she needs to be reassured that this was not her fault because it was *not* her fault. Talk to her and tell her very calmly that it is a tragedy, but there is no one to blame. She did not do anything wrong and together the two of you will study and figure out what happened so that next time, when she is ready, there will be a better outcome. Let her know that you love her and this does not change your feelings toward her. About this time she should look up at you where she has not before, looking for reassurance. Tell her, without touching her that you love her unconditionally and mean it.

The second step is to let her know that when she is ready you will be waiting to hold her. Let her know that you understand the pain she is suffering and are willing to give her a safe place to heal and regroup. When she is convinced, within her own heart that you do not blame her and are accepting of her unconditionally, she will return to you. Do not push any form of physical contact. It may take a few minutes or it may take a few days, but when she comes to terms with the situation and feels safe, she will reach out to you. Not for sex, just for loving arms.

Until she has an understanding of what happened, she may have an adverse reaction to sex. She will not want to "risk" another pregnancy until she understands what happened and how she can make sure it will not happen again. She may be cautious about lovemaking for several weeks, be patient.

To the Woman who lost the pregnancy: The loss of a pregnancy that you had your heart set on is one of the hardest things you will ever endure. Everything inside you is set up to make you bond with your child, hormone levels, upbringing, and instinct. Then to have it taken away in such a short time is devastating and you have every reason to feel sorrow, losing a baby is a tragedy.

Taking some of the amino acid GABA at 750mg doses, three times a day should help take the edge off the pain and help you deal more reasonably with your loss.

Steeping three level tablespoons of rubbed sage, (from the grocery or herb store) in a quart of hot water for tea and drinking it, can help balance the hormones and hypothalamus to help you heal, both physically and emotionally. The hypothalamus controls all involuntary actions in the body as well as playing a major role in emotions and healing from trauma.

You need to understand that even though you have experienced a hard loss, so has he. Go back to your mate and give him a loving hug and let him know that you understand that he too has had a loss and that you would like to work through things together. Unite as a team to understand what happened and then use this time to grow together.

Read through the next section to figure out what happened so you can hopefully find resolution, and lessen the chances of ever having to repeat it. See if you can find a pattern to make sense of your own situation and then work toward resolving those problems. Doing something positive will make you feel better.

Did you know that studies have shown, over 90% of women who lose a wanted pregnancy will become pregnant, again, within twelve months? Prepare now for the next pregnancy.

Troubleshooting miscarriages

These are several of the more common reasons for miscarriages and each will be discussed in this section. Miscarriages don't "just" happen and they come with signs that point to an underlying problem. If you have already had a miscarriage, then look back at the symptoms. Each miscarriage has its own profile that lets us know what is happening in the body so we can help to prevent the problem from repeating in the future. Anytime there are any signs of cramping or spotting during pregnancy it needs attention. Spotting and/or cramping are not normal signs of a healthy pregnancy. As always, at any point you are not in control then you should seek help from your health care provider.

Estrogen is a hormone in your body. In part, it affects the hypothalamus resulting in involuntary actions in the body such as emotional stability, labor contractions, firm muscle tone, nurturing instincts and milk production.

Progesterone is the balancing agent for estrogen and causes relaxation of the muscle, mental stability and slows milk production. During the first two and a half trimesters the predominant hormone should be progesterone, also considered the "pregnancy hormone". It relaxes the muscles, not only visible muscle but also internal muscles such as the uterus and the ones supporting the hips and low torso, which allows the baby to grow and allows the hips to spread so baby can move through the birth canal during labor.

An imbalance, of too much estrogen, generally begins with sore breasts, uterine cramping and/or emotional changes such as over-reaction. This happens more with, but is not limited to, larger breasted women or with a female baby because there is a higher release of estrogen that may not be balanced with adequate amounts of progesterone for a stable pregnancy. A miscarriage caused from estrogen will generally occur during the first twelve weeks of the pregnancy.

During the last month of pregnancy, a woman can generally feel the estrogen kick in as the hips spread, Braxton Hicks contractions set in, baby settles down into the pelvis, muscle tone improves, and the woman goes into 'nesting'. Not having this change in hormones could result in a delay, or failure to go into labor. By the same respect, if these things happen during the early months of pregnancy then the pregnancy could be at risk.

Breast Soreness: The first sign of a miscarriage is usually breast soreness and at this point we would insure the mother is taking one dose of Vitamin E (d-alpha) 400i.u. per day. Vitamin E is not only specific for relieving breast soreness, but it allows the body to heal without scarring, is an antioxidant, and also assists in improving oxygen assimilation.

Cramping: If cramping begins then it is immediately time to stop and pay attention. Cramping is not a natural part of pregnancy, no matter how common it may be. It would be good to start taking a natural form of progesterone to increase the relaxant properties to neutralize the excess estrogen. Sarsaparilla tea or capsules have been used, historically, for relaxing the uterus to stop cramping. Progesterone creams with 500mg per ounce of progesterone can be rubbed in to the soft skin areas of the body at ¼ tsp doses to get quick results. This is generally stopped after the cramping stops. Get off your feet and stay down.

Spotting: If spotting starts, no matter how light, I usually start my ladies on Ferrum Phos., this is a homeopathic form of iron phosphate that assists to slow bleeding. With cramping and spotting, I suggest absolute bed rest until 24 hours after the last signs of any spotting. I also suggest increasing the vitamin E to 400iu three times per day for a short time. The Vitamin E is cut back to 400iu per day as soon as the cramping has stopped. DO NOT USE ICE PACKS! Ice is going to cause the uterus to contract and that is already an instigating factor in this case.

Lifting anything over 25 pounds is inappropriate for an expectant mother and it has nothing to do with how strong her back or arms are. During pregnancy the placenta attaches itself to the uterine wall and when we lift something we tighten the muscles inside the abdomen as well as the legs, back etc. and this tightening causes the uterus to contract. The placenta, being an independent unit without muscle, does not contract. Lifting too much will cause a, usually brief, cramp followed by spotting hours later. At first it is usually brown, and dark in color, which is show of what got started from the lifting. If the bleeding increases and gets bright red then it has not healed back and the separation between the uterus and placenta continues. This can happen any time during pregnancy.

Get off your feet, and that means completely off the cervix, too. If you are sitting, the weight of the baby and uterus are still sitting on the cervix and the body is getting signals to dilate. For a flow, as opposed to a spot, a pillow can be put under the hip to bring the uterus a little above the heart, causing the heart to have to pump the blood uphill to continue a bleed. This lessens blood loss. Stay down, in a position with the heart at or below uterine level, until the placenta has a chance to heal back to the uterus, usually a couple of days.

Put an ice pack on the tummy, just above the pubic bone to cool the point of bleeding. No more than 30 minutes at a time. Cooling an area will constrict the blood vessels to reduce bleeding.

Vitamin E (d-alpha) 400iu three times per day for 48 hours can assist with healing.

Ferrum Phos. 6X can stop the bleeding and increase oxygen assimilation (this can be repeated whenever there is an increase in bleeding)

Shepherd's Purse tea (one teaspoon powder in one cup of hot water up to four cups per day) anytime bleeding increases.

Drinking at least six cups of prenatal tea per day can give nutritional support to the female organs.

If the placenta has pulled far enough off the uterus and is not able to heal back, then the bleeding will increase until the placenta is completely detached. Stay down and continue the program until the bleeding slows to avoid a hemorrhage.

If there is blood loss to a point of the lips losing color or dizziness occurs with sitting or standing then a health care professional should be immediately contacted.

Urinary tract infections: Symptoms are frequent urination, pain in the kidney region of the back, pain or burning with urination, blood or mucous in the urine, foul smelling urine. If left unattended for an extended period of time it can cause nausea, vomiting, fever, chills and possible premature labor. This can happen any time during pregnancy but it is most common in the last half of pregnancy when there is more pressure on a woman's kidneys.

Infection shows up in a urine strip as leukocytes and nitrites. If these test positive then either contact your healthcare professional or start on large amounts of high potency colloidal silver (500 to 1100ppm) and golden seal or Oregon grape every hour. If results are not showing improvement within 12-24 hours OR if the symptoms continue to worsen then seek attention immediately.

Low Blood Pressure or Anemia (low iron) Not having enough blood in the system will cause fatigue and weakness with dizziness upon rising. The problem can be from either not having enough volume (low blood pressure) or not enough iron to produce enough healthy red blood cells (anemia). Either way, spotting can be a result of inadequate blood supply.

1) Low Blood Pressure: Anything below 100 Systolic or below 60 Diastolic are considered too low for pregnancy and can result in bleeding. There can also be a heat or cold sensitivity. If this is the case then a woman's blood pressure may quickly be brought within a normal range by drinking one quart of electrolytes (recipe in the First Trimester chapter). Replacing fluid volume, by drinking electrolytes, within the body will usually show results within an hour or so. One quart per day for the week or so will usually be beneficial then the amount can be dropped back to ½ quart per day to maintain normal blood pressure levels. Again, listen to your body.

2) Anemia: If a woman is pale for her nationality, feels tired, has possible heart palpitations or shortness of breath. A rather rapid way to bring iron and vitamin K levels up is by taking a package of fresh spinach mixed with fruit or fruit juice and blending it in a blender together and then drinking it. Running it through the blender will assist with faster assimilation as it is already in a pre-digested state. Results should be seen in a couple of hours. Follow-up would include taking a ferrous sulfate supplement because it is one of the faster supplements to be assimilated without causing constipation. The usual dosage of ferrous sulfate is one per day, but can be taken in doses up to two per day, if taken separately. Along with taking this supplement, eat those greens and beets!! They are wonderful for building the blood.

Overheating (environmental or diet) Signs of excess heat in the body can range from inflammations of the eyes, ears, nose and throat, red complexion, flushed or fevered feelings and headaches to joint pain, skin eruptions and excess bleeding (such as nose bleeds, uterine bleeding, bruising, etc). Emotional signs include frustration, irritability and anger. The heat can come from being exposed to environmental heat such as sunshine or excess room temperatures. Excess heat can also be induced by eating heat producing foods such as cayenne, jalapeno, salsa or any other heat producing (hot spicy) food.

The earlier signs of miscarriage caused from overheating will usually be fatigue and bleeding (either old, brown blood or else fresh, red blood). There are usually no signs of cramping until after bleeding has started and it is usually not associated with breast soreness. It usually occurs within 24-36 hours after being over heated but can have a delayed time. It is best to avoid excess heat during pregnancy and I suggest that expectant moms stay away from heat producing foods in order to lessen the risk of this type of miscarriage. Drinking mint tea can assist in cooling the blood.

Thyroid A hypothyroid (or an under active thyroid) can cause weight gain, sensitivity to the cold, weak kidneys and/or bowels along with hair loss, depression, fatigue, memory loss, muscle aches, slow metabolism, and decreased sex drive. People who have hypothyroidism tend to have cold hands and the skin on the hip is generally cold (even in warm weather). People with hypothyroidism crave sweets, caffeine and breads, which are exactly the foods that cause them the most problems. Thyroid hormones affect every part of the body and can be a major cause of an incompetent cervix during pregnancy. Therefore premature labor is a sign of a possible thyroid issue if some of the other signs are also present.

By stopping the foods that are causing the problems and increasing the amount of protein going in, the body can help to balance the thyroid during pregnancy. Focusing on eating meats, eggs, beans and nuts and also taking two tablespoons of a unflavored gelatin supplement a day are all good ways of increasing the amount of protein needed.

Kelp is a good mineral, if it can be obtained from a clean source. It is easily assimilated and replaces all of the minerals the thyroid needs.

The best all around thyroid supplement that I have seen has 100mg of raw glandular thyroid (bovine) along with tyrosine, copper, iodine, calcium and zinc. The usual recommendation is two with breakfast and one more at lunch. Thyroid supplements should always be taken with food and should not be taken at night, as they can stimulate enough energy to cause difficulty sleeping. Note: If nausea occurs (within about 20 minutes) with the glandular thyroid then there is too much being taken or it is not needed.

Environmental toxins The most common environmental toxins are viral infections. Toxins from the environment, water, or bacteria such as E. coli can cause a miscarriage. This type of miscarriage is the hardest to stop because generally by the time there are any symptoms, a "pregnancy loss" has already taken place by a week or more. There are usually no signs of fatigue, cramping, sore breasts, etc. and there is only a loss of movement. This type of miscarriage may not even show up as an infection, on a urine strip, if the infection is isolated to the uterus and does not reach the kidneys. In this event, one should be checked so that the chemical, bacterial, or viral intruder can be neutralized prior to the next pregnancy. These kinds of miscarriages happen most often in the last two trimesters.

Sometimes an enlarged head in the fetus, from hydrocephalus, will be noted and is usually caused from bacterial of viral infections. Obvious deformations can be from chemicals or else a lack of folic acid, which assists with cell division for proper growth. There is usually some decomposition in the remains so it is difficult for a "lay" person to tell the cause. If you have a late term miscarriage (or stillborn) it would be in your best interest to have a blood test done to find the cause. You may even want to have a full autopsy for your own knowledge. This would allow you the opportunity to possibly eliminate the source.

Note: In most states it is unlawful to have a late term miscarriage or stillborn without reporting it to the state you are residing in. If a late term miscarriage were to take place outside of a facility then you would need to take the remains in for a death certificate and analysis. Meanwhile, if it happens inside a medical facility the it is presumed that all that could be done was done and there is usually no further investigation. Remember to check the laws in your state.

After Miscarriage Cleanse
1) Keep the bowels open to at least twice per day.
2) Burdock Root: is a blood detoxifier. Take two capsules of burdock root three times per day with a glass of apple juice (to assist in cleansing the liver).
3) Lobelia: Historically, lobelia neutralizes many poisons and is considered a broad base infection fighter. The herbalists of old called it the "thinking herb" as it appears to have resolved problems that they were not sure of the cause. Take one capsule three times per day with meals. (Do not take lobelia by more than one capsule per dose.)
4) Prenatal Tea: Drinking one cup of prenatal tea three times per day to nutritionally support the female organs.

This cleanse should be continued for a minimum of 30 days, taking caution to avoid getting pregnant during the next cycle (about two weeks).

Once one has determined what the cause is, the following are general recommendations I may make to my ladies.

For Viral Infection Losses:
1) After miscarriage cleanse.
2) Two yarrow capsules three times per day. More if it is a virus that tends to cause bleeding. Yarrow has been historically used as an anti-viral and helps to stop bleeding. For high blood pressure individuals Oregon grape should be used to replace the yarrow.
3) One Lobelia capsule three times per day. If lobelia causes nausea then garlic capsules should be used instead, though is not always as effective.

My most common recommendation is to take two capsules of yarrow twice a day during any pregnancy, following the miscarriage. In the occurrence of high blood pressure, then the supplement should be changed to one yarrow capsule and one garlic capsule twice a day.

For Bacterial Infection Losses: The doctor will generally recommend a run of antibiotics.
1) Follow the doctor's instructions and after completing those instructions do an After Miscarriage cleanse.
2) Follow up with 500ppm colloidal silver, one dropper three times per day and two capsules of goldenseal root three times per day for one month. After a month of taking the goldenseal root, stop taking it and continue to follow the remaining program for, at least, an additional month before getting pregnant again. Following diet will also help to strengthen the immune system.

For Chemical Exposure Losses:
1) Follow the After Miscarriage Cleanse
2) Take two Goldenseal root capsules three times per day. Goldenseal root has a history of neutralizing many types of chemicals.
3) Take one capsule of Lobelia three times per day with meals. This is a 60-90 day program prior to conceiving again.

Drugs, Alcohol or Smoking are also causes of miscarriages. These would fall under environmental toxins. It would be suggested, the cause be eliminated and the instructions below be followed before trying to get pregnant again.
1) Follow the After Miscarriage Cleanse
2) Take two Goldenseal root capsules three times per day. Goldenseal root has a history of neutralizing many types of chemicals
3) Take one capsule Lobelia three times per day with meals.
4) Follow program and diet for at least three months prior to getting pregnant again.

~~~~~A Short Story~~~~~

One day I received a call from a woman who was about seven months pregnant with her fourth child. She was bleeding and rightfully worried about losing her baby. I asked several questions trying to locate the reason for the bleed so we would know how to treat it. She had not been exposed to illness, she had not been sick, she had not fallen, she had not been around chemicals, she had not lifted anything heavy, she had not had any breast soreness or cramping. Her energy and strength was good and her color was still pink and healthy. She did not show any signs of thyroid problems or infections. She had plenty of movement from the baby.

"Hmmm, OK" I said "Tell me what you have done in the last 24 hours". (The instigating factor will usually, not always, be found within 24 hours prior to a symptom)

She thought about it a minute and then she went through her day from the morning before and in a minute she said "Wait! Would picking up the toilet have done this?"

"Yes," I replied "That could have certainly done it. Do tell me why you were lifting a toilet while you are pregnant!?"

"Well, my husband got frustrated with his job and the phone kept ringing so he flushed his cell phone down the toilet. I lifted the toilet to retrieve the phone."

To most women, lifting a toilet would be so out of character that they would not have done it at all, but this little gal was raised to be very independent and her parents had taught her to be a good worker. Moving a toolbox, three times her weight was not an issue. Pulling a toilet was a 10 minute job that was not worth thinking twice about. I have an utmost respect for hard workers, and this little gal is a keeper, but these ladies do present this type of problem more often than other women.

Our little mother laid down, took Ferrum Phos 6X, drank a cup of Shepherd's Purse tea, took 400iu Vit E, and then used ice packs on her tummy just above the hair line. In a couple of hours she had everything under control with no more signs of bleeding. She stayed down for the rest of the day and through the night. The next day she took things easy and the following day she was back to her old self. There were no problems through the rest of her pregnancy.

NOTES_____

_____

_____

_____

_____

_____

_____

_____

~10~
FIRST TRIMESTER
Most common challenges and solutions

Breast Soreness The breasts become sore and are uncomfortable, sometimes without even being touched. Though it is usually not so intense, it can be to a point that the bra or shirt are uncomfortable to come in contact with them. Generally, this is paralleled with the breasts getting larger or swelling. This is usually more common when there is a female baby due to the added production of estrogen but can occur with either of the following problems.

1) Lack of Vitamin E. Inadequate amounts of vitamin E in the body to provide for the body's needs. Vitamin E has historically been a specific for breast soreness.

Possible Solutions. Supplement Vitamin E (d-alpha) at 400i.u. per day. There should be a noticeable change within three to four days if this is the problem. Continue throughout the pregnancy as Vitamin E also has other advantages such as to prevent scarring, oxygenating the blood and is a well documented antioxidant.

Caution. Vitamin E is oil soluble so it is possible to over dose therefore the amounts should not be increased without a specific reason.

2) Lack of Progesterone: Progesterone is the predominant hormone during pregnancy. Progesterone causes relaxation of the muscles and uterus which allows the hips to spread so baby can slide down between the hips during the final weeks as well as to relax the uterus to avoid a miscarriage. Estrogen causes contractions and is important during the end stages for labor and delivery but should not be in excess during the first 2 ½ trimesters. If the breast soreness is paralleled with uterine or muscle cramps then progesterone, in some form, can be supplemented to balance the system to avoid a potential miscarriage.

Possible Solution: Two capsules of Sarsaparilla root three times per day. Sarsaparilla stimulates the body to produce more progesterone. This can usually be stopped at the end of the twelfth week. If the cramping and soreness returns upon quitting then it can be continued until the end of the 36th week of pregnancy. If used too late in the pregnancy, can delay the onset of labor. If the Sarsaparilla is not strong enough to get symptoms under control, along with Vitamin E, then progesterone creams can be purchased at many health food or nutrition stores or online. A good progesterone cream should resolve symptoms within an hour or so and will have about 500mg of progesterone per ounce and is used in doses of about ¼ tsp rubbed into any soft skin area of the body such as stomach, under the breasts, inside the arms etc. The harder skin does not absorb as well.

Caution: Do not massage the breasts, at this point, because breast stimulation causes uterine contractions and can also increase the amount of estrogen produced which can lead to a miscarriage and also cause the breasts to become more painful.

Constipation Taking longer than 12-14 hours transit time for foods to go through the system. Fewer than two bowel movements in 24 hours is a sign of constipation. Hard or firm stools also are signs of constipation.

1) Lack of Water. The human body is over 50% water. Without proper water intake many parts of the body can dehydrate, including the bowels. Water is going to be placed into primary areas first such as blood and vital organs leaving constipation to possibly be an early sign of dehydration.

Possible Solution: Drink good, clean water more frequently. The best sources are 'well' or 'spring' water from reliable sources. The next best is filtered water. I generally recommend approximately 1 quart of fluid for every 40-45lbs of body weight, per day. This includes water, unsweetened juice and herbal teas. Note: I never recommend distilled water for consumption as it is known as a 'hungry' water. The distillation process takes all the minerals and nutrients out of the water so it picks up nutrients along the way absorbing nutrients out of the body. This same process is what makes it excellent for making extracts, teas and such where we want to pull the nutrients out and suspend them in the fluid. Carbonated and sugared drinks are not considered part of the water intake.

2) Lack of Fiber. Fiber provides the bulk, or sponge like material, in the bowel as to give the stool texture and hold the bowel shape and strength.
Possible Solution: Eat more fresh, low acid fruits. Apples, melons, pears, peaches etc. Fruits are our cleansers and assist in the cleaning of the liver, kidneys and bowels. More fresh vegetables and whole grains provide extra fiber. I generally suggest our ladies eat a fresh apple each evening along with at least one fresh green salad during the day.

3) Lack of Friendly Flora. Friendly flora also known as 'friendly bacteria' or 'acidophilus' are the friendly micro-organisms that we need for proper digestive and immune function.
Possible solution: I recommend a brand that has a combination of at least eight strains of friendly bacteria with a minimum of eleven billion organisms per serving. Suggesting at least three servings per day.

4) Lack of Exercise. Bowel function requires a certain amount of hip movement type of exercise to function properly.
Possible Solution: Walk. This is especially important for those working office or cashier type jobs where they are stuck to a sitting or standing position all day. Brisk walk for no less than one mile per day. Note: Slowly walking along, with a toddler on hand, is not going to do the same thing as putting the child in a stroller and walking at a good pace.

Fatigue or Dizziness The feeling of having lack of energy and having need for naps during the day. Feeling light headed or dizzy.
1) Nutritional Deficiency: Not enough nutrition going in for the added needs of the pregnancy.
Possible Solution: High potency, natural multi vitamin and mineral combination. Combination needs to be high in B-Complex, Vitamin C and folic acid. It should also contain a balance of minerals including iron to support the added blood being produced for the baby and placenta. I like Super Supplemental with iron from Nature's Sunshine. Most common dosage is two in the morning and two at lunch.
Caution: Supplements high in B-Complex should not be taken after about 2 PM as they can keep you awake due the energy production that a high quality B-Complex gives.

2) Low Blood Pressure. Feeling dizzy / weak upon standing or when blood pressure being taken is below 100 Systolic (top number) or below 60 Diastolic (bottom number).
Possible Solution: Electrolytes. A balance of minerals and glucose with a mild acid ph to assist with cell penetration. Electrolytes play a major role in hydration, overall strength and energy and reversing low blood pressure. Following is the electrolyte recipe I use is:

ELECTROLYTES
In a quart jar mix:
1/3 cup honey
1/3 cup lemon juice OR apple cider vinegar
½ tsp. Real Salt
½ tsp. baking soda
(Continued on next page)

Stir until the foam goes down then fill the jar the rest of the way with water. In the event of low blood sugar or the amount of honey is too sweet, that amount can be cut down. Pure maple syrup can also be used for the glucose in place of the honey.

Caution: This recipe is not to be used by anyone with high blood pressure. Diabetics need to either cut back the amount of glucose (honey or maple) or leave it out completely. Note: Real Salt is a pink mined salt that, unlike modern sea salts, is free from modern day contaminants while maintaining the same stabilized mineral content as the human body, identical to ancient sea water.

3) Anemia: Lack of strong, healthy red blood cells. Usually shows up as a pale complexion for the nationality. If the lip color is pale or there is no blushing coloration across the nose and cheeks then anemia needs to be considered.

Possible solution: Ferrous Sulfate 47.5mg is a slow release iron supplement that is not prone to cause constipation and nausea the way some other iron supplements can. It is also more readily assimilated. Ferrous sulfate can be purchased at most pharmacies. Anytime an iron supplement is taken, a balanced amount of vitamin C should be taken to assist in proper absorption of the iron. There should not be a need for additional Vitamin C as there is an adequate amount in the multi vitamin and mineral supplement.

4) Inadequate Diet. Lacking the proper meats and vegetables for the needs of the body. Fruits work as cleansers while meats and vegetables are builders.

Possible solution: Make a conscious effort to eat more greens, beets and meats. Remember that the meats and vegetables are the builders that support the body for strength. Snacking between meals is perfectly acceptable as long as dietary guidelines are followed.

Flatulence Lower intestinal gas, with or without pain.

1) Lack of Digestive Enzymes: Enzymes assist in the breaking down of foods so that the foods can be properly assimilated without undo stress on the digestive system.

Possible Solution: Take a digestive enzyme supplement. When shopping for a digestive enzyme make sure to get a 'broad based' enzyme complex that assists in digesting proteins, carbohydrates, glucose, fats etc. Not one that is just for one thing or another. Try to get as much in one supplement as possible. There are many good digestive enzymes that can be purchased.

2) Inadequate Liver function: There can be pressure or pain under the right rib cage, front or back. Stool color could be light, or have a green or orange tint to it instead of a healthy brown color.

Possible solution: Ginger root capsules. I generally recommend two capsules before each meal. If using bulk ginger then one capsule would be equal to ¼ tsp. For women who are not diabetic, drinking a large glass of apple juice twice per day has been known to help stimulate the liver.

3) Improper Diet: Taking foods in that are hard on the liver that the body has to work harder to break down. Some foods that are common for stressing the liver are fried or greasy foods, chocolate, sugar and heat producing foods such as chili, jalapeno etc.

Possible solution: Change diet to eliminate the foods that are giving the liver grief. Whatever *your* body has trouble breaking down. This may be totally different than anyone else, just keep track of what you are eating and when the problem occurs. It should form a pattern.

4) Lack of Protein: Not enough protein to balance the amount of carbohydrates being ingested resulting in combustion of gas in the intestinal tract.

Possible solution: Drink two tablespoons unflavored, unsweetened beef gelatin in warm broth one or two times per day. Gelatin melts at 98F so is easier to consume warm than cold gelatin. The increase in protein should help reduce gas shortly.

Food Cravings The urge to eat specific foods. Cravings generally show a pattern which points to a specific deficiency. Most cravings can be identified into a category such as these.

1) Salty or Sea Foods: generally point to the body being deficient in balanced minerals.
Possible Solution: A good grade of colloidal minerals. Colloidal minerals are minerals that are suspended in water which makes them easier to assimilate and the molecule is small enough to not damage the liver like some others can. Generally one or two ounces per day is enough to balance the system. A high quality mineral is very tart in flavor, if the product is sweet or flavorless then it is probably diluted and going to be ineffective.

2) Dairy Products: shows a lack of calcium.
Possible Solution: Supplement the calcium with a liquid calcium containing more than one type of calcium such as Calcium Phosphate, Calcium Citrate, Calcium Gluconate, and Calcium Lactate but none should be from a rock base. A calcium that is going to be effective will usually slow the heart rate in about 15 to 20 minutes. To test your calcium to see if it is working in your system--First, take your resting heart rate. Take your calcium (usually two tablespoons) and then wait about 20 minutes and take your resting heart rate, again. The rate should be slower after the calcium. Most calcium supplements are taken at night time to help assist with peaceful rest.

3) Meat Cravings: show a lack of protein.
Possible solution: Continue the meat consumption as long as it is not pork or processed meat and is grown without hormones or antibiotics. If meats are not available, then beef gelatin is high in protein. It does, however, need to be mixed with a warm liquid as gelatin melts at 98 degrees and sets up at 97 degrees or below. Other forms of protein are eggs, block cheeses, beans and nuts but one needs more of these foods as the protein levels are not as high as that of meats.
Caution: Protein drinks or supplements with amino acid isolates have been paralleled with specific types of birth defects so do not use them.

4) Sugar Cravings: generally show a blood sugar imbalance and shows a need for more protein.
Possible Solution: Stop sugar and replace any sweets eaten with fruits, honey, agave or other natural, unprocessed sweetener. Eat plenty of nut butter, meats, nuts, eggs or any other healthy form of protein.
Caution. Protein drinks or supplements with amino acid isolates have been paralleled with specific types of birth defects so avoid those.

5) Dark Vegetables: show a need for more iron.
Possible Solution: The vegetables are good but they may be slow to take effect so ferrous sulfate supplementation may be needed. Juicing the same veggies to drink more of the vegetables than is possible to eat and putting the vegetables into a 'pre-digested' state so they are more completely assimilated.

6) Dirt: generally basement dirt, shows a lack of minerals.
Possible solution: A good grade of colloidal (liquid) minerals. Generally 1-2 ounces per day is enough to balance the system. Note: High quality colloidal minerals are generally very tart.
Caution: dry or tablet minerals can be hard for the liver to break down so should be avoided.

Frequent Urination Having to urinate more frequently than the amount of fluids ingested would ordinarily require.
1) Sugar or Carbonation Consumption: tend to weaken the bladder muscle and kidneys.
Possible Solution: Drink water and herbal teas. Avoid drinking anything with sugar, artificial sweeteners or carbonation. Honey or stevia are acceptable sweeteners that do not add to urinary weakness. Taking Cornsilk capsules or tea as it has been, historically, used to strengthen and tone

up the bladder muscle preventing urinary incontinence.

2) Urinary Tract Infections: are generally, not always, associated with painful urination and/ or pressure or discomfort above the pubic bone in the bladder or under the ribcage in the back in the kidney region.
Possible Solution: Drink plenty of water to flush the urinary tract out. Take some kind of natural infection fighter such as colloidal silver, echinacea, grapefruit seed extract. If this is not strong enough to eliminate the infection then contact your health care provider for something stronger. Urinary tract infections can lead to premature labor if left unattended.

3) Change of Amniotic Fluid: The fluid around the baby needs to change several times per day. Amniotic fluid is not stagnate water. The fluid coming off has to go through your kidneys.
Possible Solution: Support your kidneys by eating a diet that does not consist of damaging foods and drinks. You can include an herbal supplement known for 'purifying the blood' such as *pau d arco* or *taheebo*. Drink plenty of water and herbal teas.

Headaches: Pain anywhere in the head and neck area. Sometimes can be behind the eyes and disturb the vision or affect the balance.
1) High Blood Pressure: When the blood pressure rises it applies extra pressure into the head which is a frequent cause of headaches during pregnancy.
Possible Solution: Please refer to the blood pressure section which gives instructions in the Second Trimester section. Also, Wood Betony is known for relieving pressure in the head and reducing pain from headaches and strengthening the vessels in the brain.

2) Tension: Carrying tension in the neck and shoulders.
Possible Solution: Get a massage (from either husband, family member or a professional). Spend less time on the computer or with other tension causing activities. Get out and have a relaxed walk for at least 30 minutes per day, make it a point to leave all stresses and concerns behind. (Stop and smell the roses!) A cup of chamomile tea is often a good stress reliever.

3) Sinus Problems: If it is a sinus headache it will generally start in the neck and go up the back of the head and then settle in behind the eyes. If it is from sinuses then the front of the face will generally feel heavy if you lean over (like putting on your shoes) where the face is flush with the floor. This is the most frequent form of headache, overall.
Possible Solution: Stop the milk. Milk forms mucous that causes the congestion buildup in the sinuses. Drink warm respiratory tea. Different brands are sold in grocery stores or in Health Food stores. There are also colloidal silver nasal sprays that can be sprayed into each nostril to assist in resolving many infections that may be there. If this does not resolve the infection then see your health care provider for a stronger infection fighter or antibiotic.
Note: Anytime we use antibiotics, we generally follow it up with a bottle or two of high potency friend bacteria (at least eight strains with eleven billion microorganisms per serving) to replace the friendly bacteria that is destroyed by the antibiotics for healthy cleanup.

Heartburn: Acid reflux. Sensation of upset stomach, acid indigestion or burning sensation in the throat or esophagus.
1) Too Many Acids in the Diet: High acid food like coffee, tomatoes, oranges etc increase the acid level in the body, especially the stomach and digestion.
Possible Solution: Stop all high acid food and drinks.

2) Lack of Digestive Enzymes: which assist in the breaking down of foods so that the foods can be proper assimilated without undo stress on the digestive system.

Possible Solution Take a digestive enzyme supplement. When shopping for a digestive enzyme make sure you get a 'broad based' enzyme complex that assists in digesting proteins, carbohydrates, glucose, fats etc. not one that is just for one thing or another. Try to get as much in one supplement as possible. There are many good digestive enzymes that can be purchased.

3) Stomach Tension: Carrying life tensions or stresses in the stomach.
Possible Solution: Catnip/ fennel liquid supplement. This is nice to have on hand as it is also good for colicky babies, too. I like a dark, thick extract made on a glycerin base. Generally, 15 drops in a cup of very warm water will do the trick, if it is a good brand.

4) Lack of Calcium: The baby is pulling minerals out of the mother to build new little bones, teeth and organs. If there is a lack of calcium then there can be several symptoms, one of which could be excess stomach acid.
Possible Solution: Supplement the calcium with a liquid calcium containing more than one type such as Calcium Phosphate, Calcium Citrate, Calcium Gluconate, and Calcium Lactate. A calcium that is going to be effective will usually slow the heart rate in about 15 to 30 minutes. To test your calcium to see if it is working in your system--First, take your resting heart rate. Take your calcium (usually two tablespoons) and then wait about 20 minutes and take your resting heart rate, again. The heart rate should be slower after the calcium. Most calcium supplements are taken at night time to help assist with peaceful rest. NOTE: I never recommend calcium supplements from a rock base such as oyster shell, coral, bone meal, egg shell as they don't tend break down to a cellular level to give the kind of support that we need in this program. They can also be more prone to cause kidney and gall stones.

Morning sickness: Vomiting and / or nausea during pregnancy, no matter the hour of day or night. Morning sickness is not a natural part of a healthy pregnancy, however, it is common.
1) Animal Milk Consumption: We were supposed to be weaned at 18 months of age as milk is the food intended for the young of the species. Nowhere else in Nature does any animal continue to drink milk after the age of weaning. Only humans and the animals we have domesticated do that. Milk is loaded with antibiotics, infections and hormones. All of which work against us when we are trying to carry a healthy pregnancy. Our body tends to rebel milk during pregnancy more than other times of life. Based on my experience, milk consumption tends to be the primary reason for morning sickness.
Possible Solution: Stop dairy especially milk, ice cream, yogurt and soft cheeses. Block cheeses do not seem to be as responsible for this problem. When you want milk for something like hot cereal try almond, coconut or rice milk. Do not use soy due to the high content of estrogen in soy. *(read more on the reasons for no soy in the diet section.)*

2) Constipation: Having fewer than two bowel movements in 24 hours. When the old stuff cannot get out it can result in the stomach rebelling the new food coming in.
Possible Solution: Open the bowels by eating fresh fruits. Generally an apple per day is enough to do it. As a supplement, a combination with Cascara Sagrada as a primary ingredient is generally helpful. Do not take so much as to cause diarrhea but enough to have two movements per day. Watery movements are not good as they can flush nutrients out and also cause the uterus to contract. Listen to your body and take only the amount needed to open the bowels to twice per day.

3) Liver: The liver produces urobilinogin and bilirubin. If the liver does not properly produce these it can cause nausea.
Possible Solution: Taking two Ginger capsules before each meal to assist in liver function helping to relieve pressure and upset in the stomach.

4) Rebellion to the Pregnancy: This has an emotional foundation and is usually found in women who are over worked, out of work, divorced, single or older women who already have their plate full of projects and don't feel like they can take on any more. Generally it is an unplanned pregnancy.
Possible Solution: Come to terms that this baby is going to be here and you are the chosen mother. This baby needs you and your acceptance. Reprioritize your life and put this child as a primary focal point. (*Please read more on this in the 'Fears' part of the Third Trimester section and in the Single Moms section*). Also, I have found Rescue Remedy to be a great asset to those who are under this kind of stress.

5) Electrolytes: control a huge part of the water balance and electrical energy in the body. Anytime there is chronic vomiting, sweating or dehydration then one can figure the electrolytes are depleted. If the cause is from lack of electrolytes then the blood pressure will usually be on the low side.
Possible Solution: Find the electrolyte recipe and instructions in the Fatigue / Dizziness part in this section and use accordingly.

6) Lack of Food Enzymes: Enzymes are needed to assist in the digestion of all foods. Cooked foods have had all the naturally occurring enzymes killed through the heating process. Generally raw fruits and vegetables have active enzymes intact.
Possible Solution: Taking two capsules of natural food enzyme complex prior to each meal is often effective. When choosing a food enzyme one should look for a product that helps with the digestion of as many food groups as possible such as proteins, fats, carbohydrates etc. There are many brands to choose from. Try to avoid products that only work for one or two food groups.

7) Low Blood Sugar: Symptoms of low blood sugar can be dizziness, weakness, hunger between meals, irritability when hungry and headaches.
Possible Solution: More frequent and smaller meals. Focus on increasing the amount of protein in the diet as protein is Nature's way of balancing the insulin production in the body.

Notes_____

_____

_____

_____

_____

_____

_____

_____

_____

~11~
BECKY'S STORY

My experience with midwives started when I was born. I had two older brothers, but I was the first of three girls to be born at home. I grew up on a farm with a stay at home mom; healthy home cooked meals, a large garden, and old-fashioned values. These traditions were ingrained in me and in 2008; I fell in love, and married a wonderful man who had many of the same values. My husband was also born at home so it was a natural expectation that we would have a midwife when the time came to have children.

Several months after we got married, I realized that I had missed my period. When we realized that I was pregnant, I got the phone book out to look for a midwife. When I was born, my mom had to have a midwife come from Ogden, so I expected that I would have to deal with the same challenges. I was pleasantly surprised when I found out that there was a local midwife. I gave Donna Young a phone call to make an appointment and we met soon after.

At our first appointment, she introduced me to her program. Over the years she had been a midwife, she noticed similarities between women who had easy births and developed a program for other women to follow to get the same results. The program included a strict healthy diet and exercises. I had very few changes that I needed to make since I had grown up with the same health emphasis.

There were a couple of challenges that I experienced during my pregnancy. At one point, I was having sharp pains that were unbearable across the front of my belly. After a couple of days of the excruciating pain and being told by everyone that it was just a natural part of pregnancy that had to be endured, I called Donna in tears. She came to my house and in a matter of moments, she had made a couple of adjustments to my body, and the pain released immediately. I cried from relief. Donna was upset that I had not called sooner she said, that pain and discomfort were not a normal part of pregnancy. I explained that I didn't know she could do anything to relieve my pain. I never hesitated to call again!

I received a great deal of criticism from friends and family that I had decided to have my baby at home. They worried aloud that anything could go wrong and if I wasn't in the hospital, I could lose the baby, or my life. They criticized the fact that I had only gained a total of six pounds during my pregnancy. Despite all of the well-meaning advice that I received, as my pregnancy progressed, I didn't share their concerns, I looked good and I felt good. Donna's program that I followed focused on recognizing and preventing possible problems before they became a problem instead of trying to deal with the problem once it was out of control. She closely monitored my body for signs of sickness or problems. The moment she became concerned with something, we took measures to correct the issue. Health experts preach that pregnant women should gain an average of thirty pounds to be healthy. I was grateful to learn that Donna's belief and studies showed that with a healthy pregnancy you would not gain unnecessary weight!

I was active up to the time I went into labor. The day I was due, I was helping my husband with yard work and repairing the sprinkler system.(*See picture-pg. 77*) At almost two weeks overdue, I was helping with branding and dehorning calves.

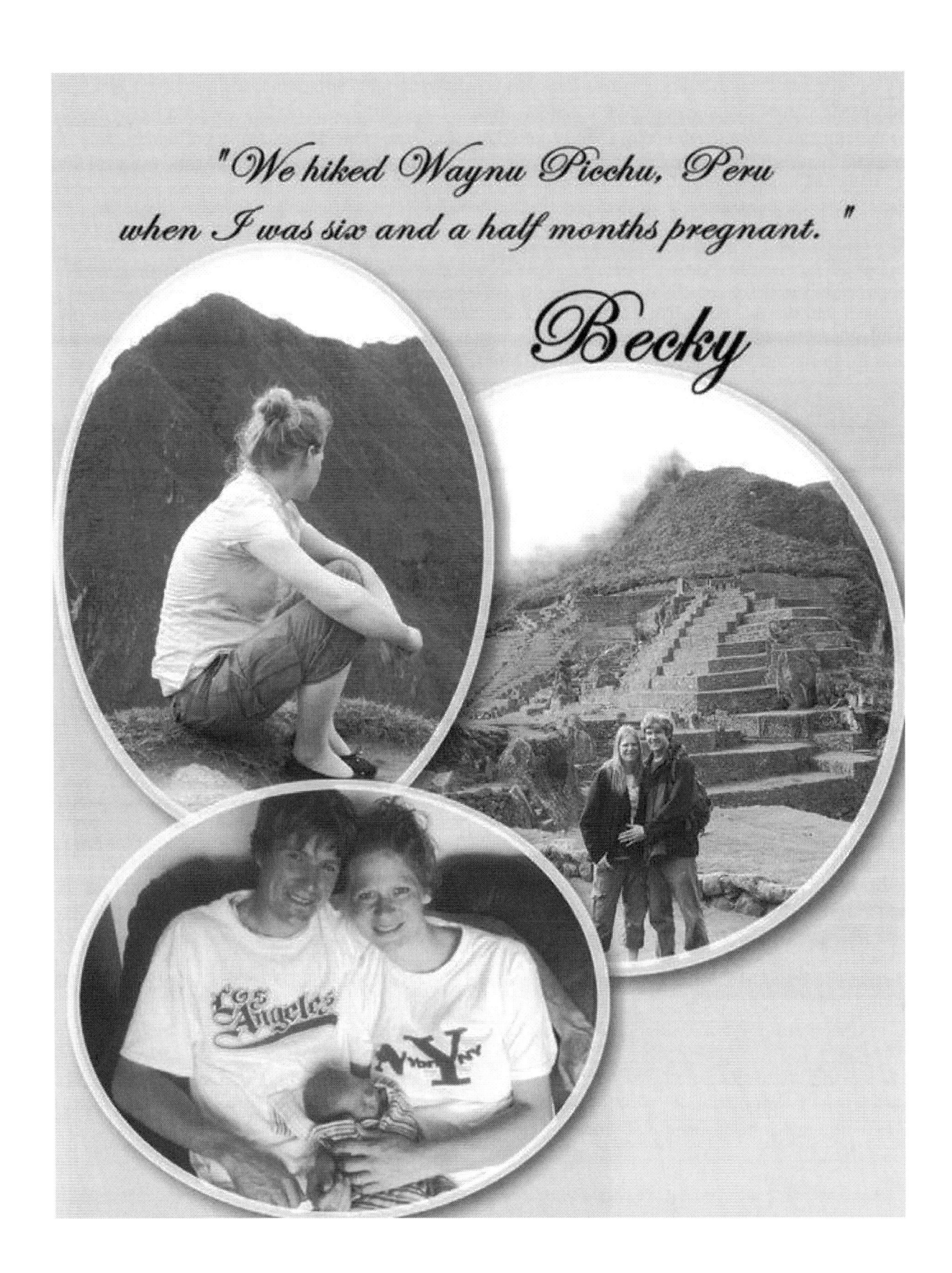

"We hiked Waynu Picchu, Peru when I was six and a half months pregnant."

Becky

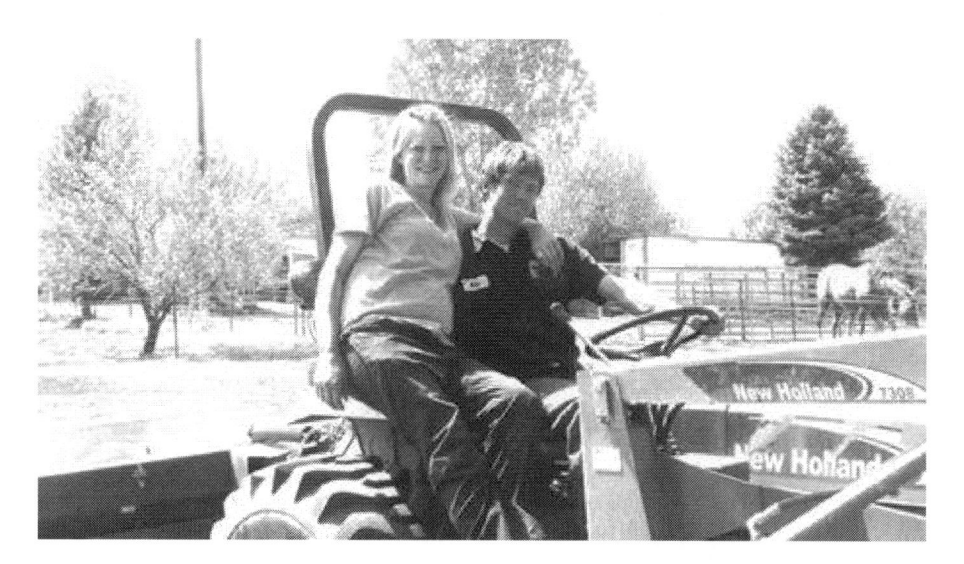

Early the next morning, my labor pains started. Donna arrived and knew exactly what needed to be done. In her competent care, I gave birth to a healthy eight pound twelve ounce baby boy that measured twenty inches long without a single tear. My birthing experience was calm and peaceful. I felt comfortable in my own home, and was able to shift positions to get more comfortable. Donna had many techniques that helped to relieve pain, tension, and fatigue. After giving birth, Donna showed me what to do to help my body to heal and return to normal. My uterus contracted to its regular size in two days, I had more milk than a Jersey cow, without ever dealing with soreness, my baby boy, Joshua's, cord fell off in three days, I only had two stretch marks, one of which had shown up the day before I gave birth, and the few hemorrhoids were gone in a week, after following instructions.

Donna had given instructions for procedures to follow that made the delivery and the days following labor go smoothly. I was able to relax and enjoy time with my sweet baby boy. After I gave birth, I felt good, and fit right back into my high school jeans that I wore six years earlier! My mom asked, after Joshua was born, "Where was Donna when I was having babies?"

Donna's program is a common sense, health based approach to childbirth that is superior to even traditional midwifery. I was grateful that I didn't have to go through a horror story to find a good experience.

~12~
SECOND TRIMESTER
Most common challenges and solutions

Dry skin is from a lack of moisture or oils in the skin causing dryness and flaking, sometimes can be itchy.
1) Insufficient Water Consumption: causes dryness throughout the system including dry skin, constipation and signs of dehydration.
Possible Solution: Drink more water as dryness generally shows lack of moisture. I generally recommend consuming about 1 quart of water (or herbal teas) for every 40-45 lbs of body weight. A 120lb person would consume about 3 quarts per day.

2) Lack of Essential Fatty Acids: Fatty acids play a major role in hair, skin and nail strength as well as muscle strength and cervical dilation.
Possible Solution: Increase consumption of foods that are high in essential fatty acids (omegas) such as fish, avocados, olive oil, nuts, seeds and chicken.
Supplement with Evening Primrose Oil. Usual dosage during the second trimester is two 1300mg soft gel-caps twice a day. There are other essential fatty acids and omegas but this one tends to be absorbed faster than most and it is specifically balanced for women's health especially cervical dilation and skin.

3) Potassium Deficiency: Potassium assists the body in balancing body fluids from the cell level all the way out to the skin. Potassium is also important in cell metabolism as well as repair and growth in the body.
Possible Solution: Eat foods high in potassium such as cabbage, carrots, bananas and celery. Taking a good potassium supplement can help balance the moisture in the body. Where sodium assists in putting nutrients into the cells, potassium assists in removing fluids off the cells. The one I generally use is a potassium citrate and potassium aspartate combination at one capsule two times per day. A little more than usual recommendations because there is more need during pregnancy....also noted that one capsule is three percent of the daily value.

Edema / Water Retention: Swelling in the body, generally starting in the feet and hands. Watch for early signs by checking to see if there are marks around the leg where the sock goes. If the sock is leaving an impression there is probably some water retention going on. Rings not fitting are another sign of water retention. All water needs to be transported out through the kidneys. If the kidneys are not transporting water out of the body then the water is stored in the body, and swelling will start being noticed in the extremities. If water retention problems are not taken care of then high blood pressure can occur.
Possible Solution: Diet. Stop taking in the things that are compromising the kidneys such as sodium chloride (table salt), sugar, carbonation (yes even that 'just one soda a week?" one), and high acid foods like oranges, grapefruit etc.

Use the Cabbage Soup recipe as outlined in the 'High Blood Pressure' section, which has been historically used to run excess fluids off the system through the kidneys and bowels.

Take a supplement that is made to work as a diuretic such as a juniper, cornsilk, dandelion combination to assist in nutritional support for liver and kidney function. Take at breakfast and lunch, do not take at night as it may keep you awake going to the bathroom.

Emotions (Nesting)   During pregnancy a woman usually becomes more emotional. Once you understand the cause of the emotion then it is much easier to deal with. The hormonal change in a woman during pregnancy, and more so in the days immediately prior to giving birth, are for the purpose of securing the environment for her child. She will want the ones she loves and trusts to be close to her. If she cannot be with the ones she loves then she will become more emotional. She wants the security of having a safe place for her new child to be born into which is very instinctive. Those who make her defensive will be pushed back.
Possible solution: Recognize the fact that what you really need is security. Sometimes we rely on others, when the one we really need to trust in is ourselves. Once you realize that you are the one responsible for your child then the privilege of being a new parent becomes easier. Look at what needs to be done to secure the environment for your new little one. The needs are simple and listed here.

Love: is easy, as soon as you look into this baby's eyes you will fall in love because you will see unconditional love in those eyes for you. Relax and let yourself go. As long as there is no selfishness, then love flows naturally. Selfishness is the only enemy to love.
My favorite part of the birth is that first eye to eye contact between mother and child. When they look into each others eyes and realize 'this is the person who loves me so much!'.

Roof Overhead: this baby will stay right there with you. No matter what your circumstances this baby will be happy anywhere you are. Baby does not care what your status is as long as you are there with gentle love and baby is fed and changed regularly then baby is happy. Clean environment is a matter of respect for you and your child. Keep things neat and in order. No matter how humble the surroundings, cleanliness is a must. Personal hygiene and a clean home are important to everyone's self esteem. For both you and baby.

I remember delivering a baby for a couple who lived in a 20 foot camp trailer. They were just starting out and it was what they could afford. He worked all day and she was home alone. They had very few belongings but everything they had, she kept neat and tidy. She cooked every meal from scratch and crocheted doilies and other crafts to add beauty to their home, she never had idle time. When he came home from work she had a wholesome dinner on the table so they could have their meals together. She was 19 years old and never felt sorry for herself for not having better things, just spent time taking care of what they had so their baby had a clean and loving home to be born into. They were both happy as they worked together to provide for their family. A couple of years later, I delivered a second baby for them in a newer and bigger home but still maintaining the same caliber of cleanliness she always had.

Blankets and Clothes: Baby will need clothes and blankets. They can be bought, borrowed or made. Blankets have been made from rags since biblical times. Make sure everything is clean and in a place set aside for your baby.
One of my greatest treasures is the blanket Grandmother made for my father and he was raised with. It was on his bed throughout his childhood years. He gave it to me a couple of years before his death, the blanket was then almost 80 years old. The pieces of material were from shirts, blankets and pants that were not able to be patched anymore in the 1920's. She told him stories of where the pieces of material came from. He told of the many nights he lay under that blanket and felt blessed that his mother cared enough to put forth the effort and love that went into making that blanket. Dad always loved 'gifts from the heart' and preferred a handmade card to a store bought one any day. A blanket you make for your child will mean as much in the years to come.

Stay busy and don't expect someone else to make you secure. Do your part and it will relieve the pressure and stress off from you as well as those around you. As you see progresses the emotions will probably be less prevalent.

Take supplements to relieve stress. Chamomile or Catnip teas are excellent to make one feel more relaxed without causing fatigue or sleepiness. Gaba 750mg capsules have also been successfully used to bring more peace of mind. One each morning is generally enough but can be taken up to three times per day.

To the Mate: When you come home, she is probably going to want some close one-on-one time from you. This is a compliment to you as it shows you are the one she trusts to be close to for security. Spend a little time each day just being close and letting her know that you love her and together all will be well. Listen to her and help her provide for her needs. Be supportive and pleasant.

Gestational Diabetes is a sign there are too many wrong types of carbohydrates going into the system. Sugar, artificial sweeteners, concentrated glucose cause the pancreas to over react (causing low blood sugar i.e hypoglycemia). After a time of over reacting then it tires and stops producing insulin, resulting in diabetes. Insulin is the balancing agent for the glucose being consumed. When the body is producing inadequate amounts of insulin then glucose will be found in the urine.

Some women do not show 'symptoms' of gestational diabetes, however others may suffer from excessive thirst or hunger, excessive urination and / or recurrent vaginal infections. The healthcare provider should pick up on clinical symptoms such as excess weight gain, increased fundal measurement, blood pressure increase and / or elevated glucose in routine urine tests.

Risks to gestational diabetes are serious, ranging from excessively large babies (generally over 9 ½ lbs), baby can be born with hypoglycemia (low blood sugar), jaundice or respiratory problems. It is a primary cause of babies being stillborn or dying in infancy.
1) Poor Diet: Too many carbohydrates in the diet.
Possible Solution: Adhere to diet more closely. Don't put in so many carbohydrates. Though corn, fruits (including juices) and potatoes may not generally cause diabetes they can certainly add to an already existing condition. Back off those as well as the concentrated sugars. Increase the amount of meats, beans, eggs, nuts and unsweetened gelatin in your diet.

2) Pancreas not Producing Insulin
Possible Solution: Drink one quart of water for every 40lbs of body weight per day. This includes herbal teas. An herbal supplement with the first two ingredients being Juniper (or Cedar) and Golden Seal root can be taken. Recommendation is usually two or three capsules three times per day for two weeks then adjust as needed.

Note: If you cannot get this under control in a short amount of time (1-2 weeks) then you need to get assistance from a healthcare provider as the risks are too great. You should see quick results if directions are followed. The blood sugar levels should begin dropping within 48 hours of changing diet and taking supplements. Not getting results means you need extra help.

Hemorrhoids are a sign of weakened circulation, below the waist, resulting in a varicosity in the rectal wall. Signs can be a noticeable protrusion outside the rectum or there can be fresh blood in the stool.
1) Constipation: is the failure to have two bowel movements per day to eliminate toxins from food that has been eaten 14 hours or more prior. Part of constipation can include a thick or hard stool that is hard to pass. These hard stools can damage the rectal wall.

Possible Solution: Get the bowels open to two or three times per day. (*See instructions for this in the First Trimester section under 'Constipation'.*)

2) Weak Circulation: in the lower part of the body.
Possible Solution: Butcher's Broom Root (scientific name--*Ruscus aculeate* --very important to check, not all Butcher's Broom are the same). I generally suggest three capsules three times per day with meals. Along with extra colloidal minerals, to support the circulation and strengthen the vessel wall. Also, if needed, one can add in White Oak bark as an astringent at two capsules three times per day.

3) Standing or Sitting in One Place for Extended Periods: is very hard on the rectum and pelvic floor.
Possible Solution: Get more exercise and try to avoid extended periods in one spot. Try to take breaks to walk around.

4) Lack of Protein: can cause hemorrhoids due to the muscle in the bowel weakening.
Possible Solution: Try drinking two tablespoons of unflavored, unsweetened beef gelatin in warm fluid twice per day. If this is the problem then signs of improvement should be noted in the first week or so.

High Blood Pressure Checking the blood pressure tells us when we have too much fluid in the system. The veins are the blood vessels that take the blood from the body back to the right side of the heart. The arteries are vessels that take the fresh blood from the heart out to the body. The blood pressure is measuring the amount of pressure against the vessel wall during different phases of the heart beat. The top number (Systolic) tells how much pressure there is against the vessel wall during the time the heart is pumping. The bottom number (Diastolic) tells how much pressure is against the vessel wall when the heart is at a resting point, between pumps.

With too much pressure, we risk heart attacks or strokes because the excess pressure is constant on the vessel wall causing a weakening or breaking down of the vessel tissue leading eventually to an aneurysm somewhere along the path...usually in the heart or brain. Too little pressure causes weakness and poor circulation resulting in fatigue and dizziness as well as increasing the chances of shock or a hemorrhage during the delivery.

When the cuff is placed around the arm and pumped up it applies pressure on the veins and arteries in the arm, just above the elbow. Adjusted snuggly with the arrow (or line) pointing to the primary blood vessel inside the elbow. (This can be found by locating the pulse point) A stethoscope is put on the vessel (pulse point) at the inside of the elbow. The cuff is pumped up to around 140 and then listened to, if a pulse is detected then pump a little higher. Locate the top number by finding the highest point a pulse can be detected through the stethoscope then allow it to feather down slowly with the bottom number being the last number there is a pulse heard.

Blood pressure over 140 Systolic or 80 Diastolic is considered high blood pressure. It is dangerous for a woman with higher blood pressure to go through the intensity of child birth because the blood pressure rises more during times of stress or pain. Ladies, who faithfully follow this diet, rarely have high blood pressure but those with high blood pressure are not qualified for home birth. Transport is expected if the systolic reaches 160 or the diastolic reaches 100.
1) Compromised Kidneys: Excess fluid in the system is generally caused because the kidneys have been compromised.
Possible Solutions: Stop all carbonation, sugar, high acid foods, pork and heat producing foods.

The following recipe is an altered version of the old recipe used for heart patients for rapid weight loss prior to surgery, to bring down blood pressure and reduce edema. Historically, I have recommended this recipe for anyone with high blood pressure to bring it down quickly and safely in most cases by opening the kidneys and directing the fluid buildup through the kidneys.

Cabbage Soup

Take a large stock pot, like a 7 quart canner cooker and put in each of the following ingredients that have been washed and finely chopped:

1 large head cabbage
1 large green pepper
1 bunch of long stemmed green onions
1 bunch celery

Once the vegetables are in the pot, fill with water to within 3 inches of the top (to allow room for boiling). Place on the stove and bring to a boil. Allow the soup to boil, covered, for at least an hour. We want all of the nutrients to be leached out of the vegetables and put into the water. Once the vegetables are thoroughly cooked to a very tender state and have lost their bright color, strain the liquid off and throw away the dead vegetables.

Drink ½ gallon of the cabbage broth per day along with eating ½ medium watermelon per day. Preferably a watermelon with seeds and the seeds are also consumed as they are a well known diuretic in their own right. Generally there is a notable drop in the blood pressure in the first 24-48 hours.

(*For Low Blood Pressure see Fatigue and Dizziness in First trimester section*)

2) Stress: can raise the blood pressure both short term and long term. In other words, if there is a stressful issue that lasts for thirty minutes or so then it is expected that the blood pressure will rise for that time and then go back down. If there is an on going stress such as finances, work or family issues then the problem can become long term.
Possible Solution: Locate the trigger point for the stress and try to get it resolved. Also, taking a supplement for stress such as calcium, chamomile or catnip may be a good plan.

3) Lack of Oxygen: can raise the blood pressure.
Possible Solution: is Co-Q-10 in a 100mg softgel which is always taken sublingually (dissolved under the tongue) and not in a powder, capsule or tablet form. Co-Q-10 is often used to increase the amount of oxygen in the blood and results could be seen within a few minutes after taking the supplement. Note: Chlorinated water can decrease the amount of oxygen in the body and if this is a problem then changing to bottled water (without chlorine) should be a viable choice.

Infections can include bacterial, viral or yeast infections.
1) Bacterial Infections: are common. They are usually associated with heat and discomfort in the originating area. They also compound and will usually get worse if left untreated resulting in fever. On a urine test bacterial infections will usually show up as nitrites and leukocytes.
Possible Solutions: For bacterial infections we generally use Colloidal Silver 1100ppm at two droppers three times a day along with a Goldenseal root and Echinacea combinations. Remember Goldenseal is not intended for long term use as it can drop the blood sugar level so is not intended for anyone who is hypoglycemic.

2) Viral Infections generally run parallel with body aches. They most frequently present in the respiratory or digestive systems and will run a course of several days and then go away on their own if untreated. The time and severity can often be cut down by treating with herbal treatment

and a clean diet. Some viral infections have been connected to specific birth defects so it is best to treat them if possible.
Possible Solution: Viral infections respond better to Yarrow, which has a historical use for viruses, especially those viruses that may cause thinning of the blood or bleeding. Yarrow is high in vitamin K and also assists in strengthening the blood. Yarrow is given as part of the pregnancy program if the mother-to-be has been exposed to viruses with rashes or has a history of late term miscarriages or stillborns caused from viral infections. **Caution**: Yarrow should never be taken by anyone with high blood pressure. Garlic or Oregon Grape would be acceptable replacements.

3) Yeast Infections: are caused from fungi and are fed by sugars, milk and flour products. They most commonly show up as vaginal infections, acne or skin irritations but are also possible in the sinus, eyes and ears as well as the bowels. They rarely have any fever associated.
Possible Solution: Diet is a must. Stop ingesting any foods that are causing the problem such as sugars, breads and milk products. Grapefruit seed extract liquid is good for most yeast infections but must always be diluted. This one tastes terrible but is usually pretty effective.

Restless legs are the sensation of discomfort or pain in the legs that prevent the legs from powering down into a restful state. This is usually noticed when we try to go to sleep or stay in a sitting position for extended periods. Restless legs are usually caused from one or more of the following issues.
1) Stimulants: If the energy from stimulants is affecting the bowel at bedtime then the legs will not relax. Stimulants can be anything from caffeine to sugar etc. Constipation or toxins in the bowel can lead to congested lymph nodes. The lymphatic system carries the toxins out of the tissues to the sources of elimination. A blockage anywhere along this path can increase problems with restless legs.
Possible Solution: Stop putting stimulants into your system. Even B vitamins should not be taken late in the day. Open the bowels to two or three times per day. Not loose, just enough to keep the toxins out of the lower extremities. Over 4 times per day is flushing out friendly bacteria and enzymes. One in the morning and one in the evening is perfect.

2) Lack of Exercise: can cause part of the problem. If the lymphatic fluid in the legs becomes stagnate then it triggers pressure in the nerves.
Possible Solution: Try going for a walk in the evening before bed. The walking will help activate the lymphatic system. This is especially important if you have a job that requires sitting, or standing in one place for hours at a time. Aerobics, sports, jogging, walking are all positive activities that put circulation into those legs. Rubbing the legs down with lotion and lavender oil has been known to help with draining the lymph nodes and relaxing the legs. 10 drops lavender oil with a lotion carrier and rubbed into each leg is enough to show relief most of the time.

Varicosities are caused from a weakening in the valves or the walls of the veins resulting in swelling and pain in the veins. The signs are soreness in the legs and swollen or broken veins in the lower extremities. These are important to recognize because, not only can they be painful and restrictive, but if the veins in the legs are weak so might be the ones in the uterus and birth canal which would increase the potential for hemorrhaging at the birth. This includes spider veins as well as varicose veins and hemorrhoids.
1) Lack of Exercise: can increase the damage of varicosities. Sitting or standing for extended periods are a primary cause of varicose veins.
Possible Solution: If you are strong enough, walk for a mile or more daily. A brisk, uninterrupted walk will increase circulation throughout the entire body. An increased oxygen rate will improve most people's health especially that tiny baby inside. Walking assists the kidney and bowel function, relieves pressure in the lower extremities by increasing circulation and oxygen as well as

pumping the lymphatic system resulting in less pressure in the legs. Sometimes when a person first starts walking it hurts for the first ¼ mile, or so, as the lymphs open up and the pressure releases and then the walking is more comfortable. The increase in circulation and the reduced edema assists in relieving pressure off the veins. Note: For those unable to walk for longer distances at a time, maybe walking for 30 minutes, as briskly as you can would help. Swelling should leave starting from the feet and then moving upward as it travels out through the kidneys.

2) High Blood Pressure: applies extra pressure on the vessel walls and adds to the discomfort and damage of the varicosities.
Possible Solution: If the blood pressure is lowered there is less pressure on the veins. Follow instructions to reduce high blood pressure in this section. These instructions should also assist in kidney and liver function.

3) Poor Circulation: in the lower part of the body can add to varicosities.
Possible Solution: Take supplements that have been historically used to support the circulation and vein strength in the lower extremities. Butcher's Broom (make sure the scientific name is Ruscus aculeate) is a staple for strengthening the veins, reducing inflammation and increasing circulation below the waist. Three capsules three times per day is generally sufficient. Note: Horse Chestnut is commonly used for varicosities but is unacceptable for use during pregnancy because it is known to thin the blood which could induce a hemorrhage during labor and deliver. <u>Do Not Use Horse Chestnut During Pregnancy.</u>

4) Lack of Assimilated Minerals: can increase the chances of weak vessels.
Possible Solution: Taking one ounce of colloidal minerals, unsweetened or flavored, per day can help. Minerals used by the ounce are generally sold in a quart size container as opposed to a dropper bottle. Improvement should be noted within the first week and the supplement is generally continued until after the birth.

Weight gain is when there is weight being stored in the body that is beyond the needs of the body and pregnancy. Quality weight gain should consist of the weight for a healthy baby, placenta and water (amniotic fluid) but anything beyond that is extra weight that the mother will either have to lose later on or else live with. Excess weight gain causes many problems during pregnancy, delivery and postpartum. During pregnancy excess weight can raise the blood pressure, reduce strength and stamina, increase depression, varicosities and toxemia to name a few. It can cause longer labors and deliveries, increase chances of a hemorrhage as well as an inability to get into comfortable positions for birthing. After the birth, excess weight contributes to postpartum depression and inhibits the healing process.
Possible Solutions: Follow diet faithfully and exercise daily. Eat more proteins, veggies, fruits and drink plenty of water and herbal teas. The culprits are probably flour, sugars and / or carbonation. Remember that it is not the quantity of food that matters it is the quality of food one should be focusing on. Eat until you are full, staying within the suggested guidelines. (*See Diet section*)

~~~~~A Short Story~~~~~

I was standing in the checkout line at the grocery store one day and looked up to see a client, in her second trimester, with her husband in the store. Standing there thinking about what a cute couple they were when all of a sudden she reached up and bit him on the cheek and pulled back about three inches and then let it snap back. "Ouch!" I thought. Just then he looked up and saw me standing there and pointed me out to her. After paying, I walked over to where they were waiting. "How often do you bite him like that?" I asked her. She blushed and said "I don't know why I do it, sometimes I just cannot resist and I want to bite him. I love it!" I recommended she start on calcium at two tablespoons twice a day and I would see them at their next appointment. Two weeks later, at their appointment, he stated that she had not bitten him in over a week and he was very grateful for the recommendation. She said she had not even tried to quit, the desire to bite just went away.

NOTES

~13~
EDELWEISS' STORY

Being the oldest of twelve kids and the only one born in a hospital. Homebirth was nothing new to me. I asked mom if I could watch her give birth and she told me that I could when I got older. When I turned eleven she said that I was old enough to witness her give birth. I helped my dad deliver my brother and it was a scary experience for me. My mom yelled, screamed, and cursed. Towards the end she got up off the bed and tried to leave the room three times. She said, "I am not doing this anymore, I am done." My dad's reply was, "Yes, we have to deliver the baby, lay back down." It was a painful birth for my mother, my brother got stuck in the birth canal and I was so scared that something was wrong. After my brother was born my dad told me, "Rub your mom's belly and rub it hard". She tried to pull my hand away because it was hurting her and I started to rub softer, but my dad again told me, "Rub as hard as you can or the placenta won't come out". As soon as she delivered the placenta my dad cut a piece off of it and mixed it in the blender with some juice and my mom then drank it. When I asked why this was done I was told that it was to prevent mom from getting an infection. I went on to help deliver four other siblings and I loved helping.

When I was 23, I met the love of my life and five months after we were married we found out that we were expecting our first baby. I knew that I wanted to have a home birth, but my husband was not raised the way that I had been and he was worried about the safety of homebirth. It took him a while, but he finally agreed to a homebirth, as long as we had a 'back-up-doctor'. I went to a doctor for all of my pre-natal care with the hopes of giving birth at home.

I spent the first four months "sick as a dog". I threw up everything that I ate and I could barely get out of bed. I called my mom, hoping that she would have a remedy, her only reply was, "Morning sickness, is just a part of pregnancy". She told me that it was a good sign to be sick and that it meant that the baby was healthy. The morning sickness did end, but the fatigue followed me throughout the rest of my pregnancy.

Six weeks before my due date I got a rash called PUPP, it was like having hives from my neck down to the soles of my feet. I was so miserable and itchy that I could not sleep. I would sit on my hands just to get through the day and I even tried putting socks on my hands to control myself from ripping my skin off. If having a rash wasn't bad enough, my face was covered in pimples, I had facial hair and my lower back ached all of the time. Needless to say long car rides were torture.

I thought even with all of the problems I was experiencing I was healthy. I ate healthy, exercised five days a week, and gained 30 pounds. I believed that in order to have a healthy baby I needed to gain 25 to 30 pounds and I thought that I was "right on the money".

I went into labor at 7:00 a.m. and was very excited to finally give birth and be able to feel comfortable in my own body again. I was fully dilated by noon and thought to myself, "This will be a fast delivery". I got down into a squatting position and started pushing and pushing and pushing... I pushed for 13 hours and still there was no baby. I was tired, very tired and this is when my husband took me to the hospital where I pushed for another hour before the doctor realized that something was wrong. My baby was posterior and she had her head cocked back in such a way that she was stuck! There was no way to get her out without causing damage to her face and this resulted in a c-section. A total of 22 hours of drug free labor, to have it all end in a c-section. When it was all over the doctor informed me that I would have to give birth in a special room, with all my future births, where they could do an emergency c-section because I was now "at

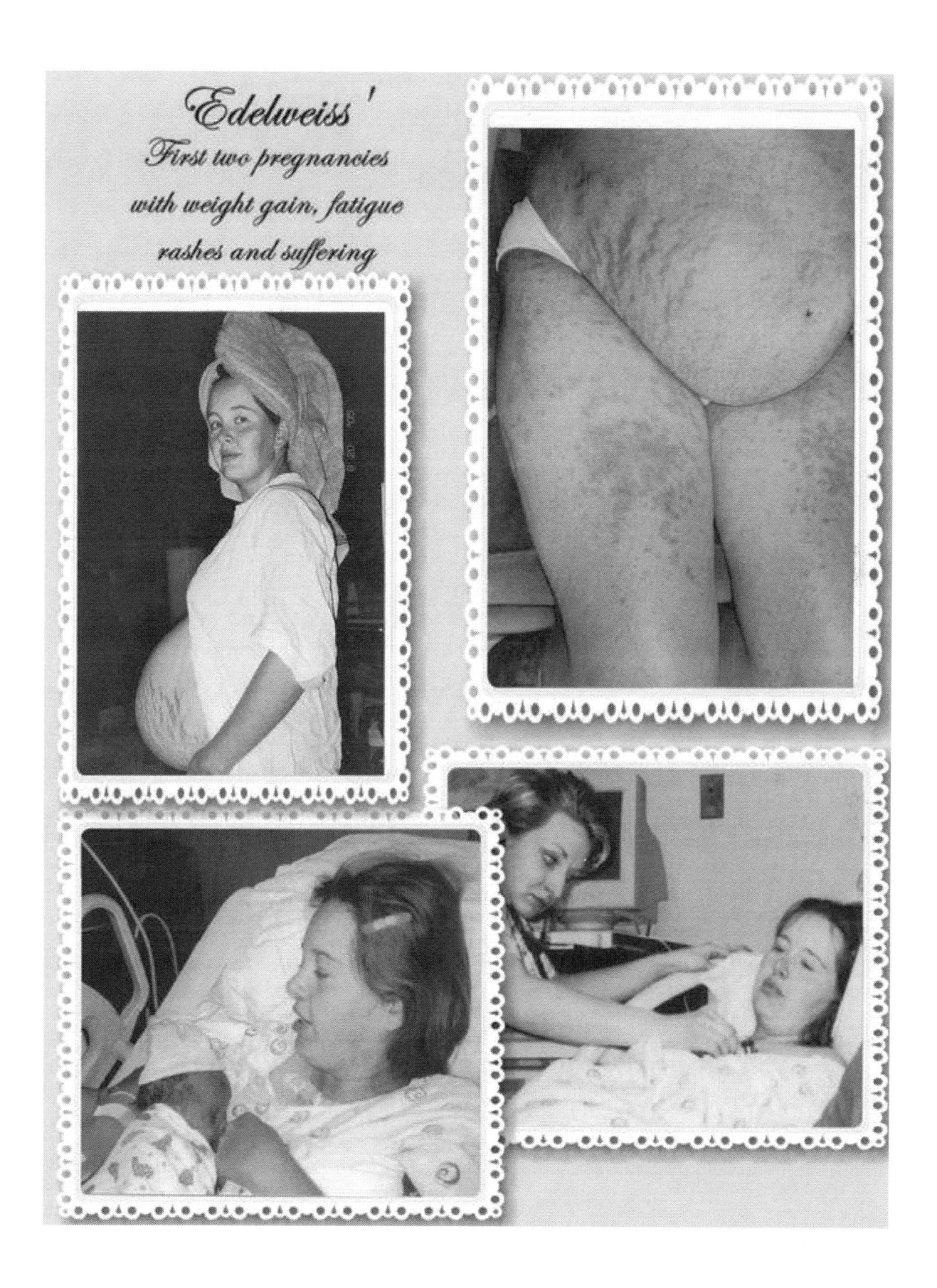

'Edelweiss'
First two pregnancies with weight gain, fatigue rashes and suffering

risk". I was completely crushed. The only thing that made the experience tolerable was my sweet baby girl, who was actually too much baby for me at 7lb 10oz.

Three months later I found out I was pregnant again and this time I didn't even dare to attempt a homebirth. I tried to eat healthy once again, but this time I felt deep down inside that it did not matter what I tried to do, I would not be able to change the outcome. Once again I got the facial hair, pimples, fatigue, and an aching back. I gained 35 pounds and you could see it in my face. It was hard to be pregnant and chase around my first baby.

With my second pregnancy I lived in fear that my dream for an all natural birth would never come true. In order to avoid being forced into another c-section I decided to show up at the hospital at the latest moment possible. So after 3 hours of excruciating labor, we left for the hospital. On the way to the hospital I had contractions that were overpowering and I screamed louder than I have ever screamed in my whole life. The contractions were more than I could handle. The minute we arrived at the hospital I was in so much pain. I walked into the lobby with only a shirt and underwear on. I did not care who saw me I felt like I was dying. My baby was coming so fast that they did not have time to prepare a room for me. They took me into a closet and laid me down on what looked like a cot and told me to push. Laying flat on my back I struggled to get up. As I was fighting to get comfortable I was met with hands forcing me to stay flat on my back. I was filled with panic. My baby's heart rate started to drop and the doctor had to pull him out using suction. I felt as though I had been raped. As soon as my son was born I asked to hold him and was told that my son needed to go to the nursery first. Once a room was ready I was moved from the closet to a room. It was an hour later and I had still not seen my son. I sat in that room and cried. My body was shaking violently and I felt as though I was laying in a bed of ice water. Not to mention that my son had just been ripped from my body. I finally walked to the nursery to see my son. When I arrived I asked to breastfeed my baby and was told that they had tubed him so he would not be hungry. I returned to my room feeling completely devastated. This was far from the birth I had wanted.

When my son was two months old, I saw an advertisement in the paper about a new midwife in town. I called her the very next day and told her that I was not pregnant, but the next time I was, I would like to use her services. The first time that I met with Donna Young, she had a calm peace about her and I liked her right off. As soon as I did get pregnant with my third baby I started prenatal care with Donna, using her technique. She taught me how to eat healthy during pregnancy, which was something I only thought that I knew. My third pregnancy was the best of my three pregnancies. I didn't have the facial hair, pimples, back pain, and I gained a healthy 17 pounds. I slept through the night up until I gave birth and learned that pregnancy did not have to feel like a death sentence. I learned that pregnancy could be an enjoyable experience.

My labor was two and a half hours and I felt like I was on top of the contractions even though I carried the fear from my first two births, and didn't completely surrender to my body. My baby weighed six pounds even, which was just right for me. I was able to get up right after having her and it was great. I was shocked at how little I bled (I have had periods that were worse). My recovery was fast and I felt so good that Donna had to keep reminding me that I had just given birth and to take it easy.

Edelweiss
With babies 3, 4 and 5
Healthy & Happy!

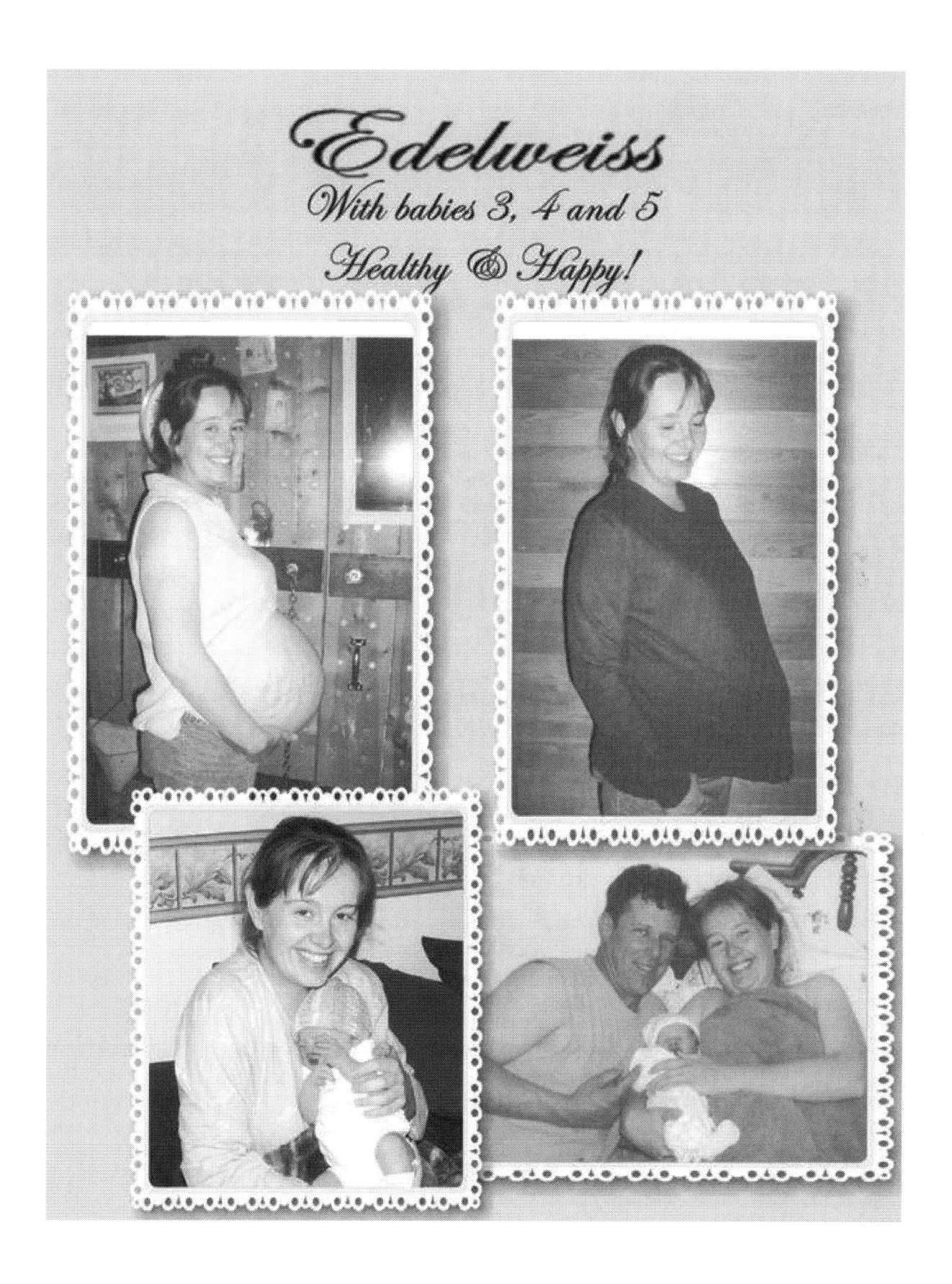

When I got pregnant with my fourth baby there was no question in my mind as to how and with whom I would deliver my baby. I thought that my third pregnancy was good, but the fourth proved to be even better. I was walking better than ever before and I knew I had to overcome the fear I had with the first two births, so that I would not carry fear into this birth. I used self hypnosis with my fourth baby and continued to stay faithful to diet and it all paid off. Once again I gained a healthy 17 pounds and I was healthier than I had ever been.

I got up to use the restroom at 12:20 a.m. when I felt a trickle of water running down my leg. Light cramps followed and I sat at the edge of the bed almost in a trance. I felt a complete calm come over me. I was relaxed and never felt like the contractions were overpowering. Donna told me that an hour had passed since my water broke (I was shocked) it felt like only ten minutes had passed. Soon it was time to push, I fell back into the old habit of trying to rush things along, I know that things would have gone better if I would have let my body do what it needed to do. Things still went great and my baby was born at 2:08 a.m. after a one hour and forty minute labor. When it came time to deliver the placenta I went back to focusing on letting my body do what it had to do and this made it the best I had ever had. The fear was gone. I was able to dress my baby, sitting up, one hour after delivery. I felt great and had a fast recovery.

Diet has helped not just with pregnancy, but with nursing too. I was not near as sore, as I was in the past, my baby seemed to be healthier, and there was no diaper rash. The only time that my baby had diaper rash was when I ate an ice cream cone, this made a believer out of me. I did not want to do anything that would hurt my little ones, so getting an ice cream cone was no longer a temptation. When my baby was four months old I was only two pounds away from the weight I was when my husband and I married. My face is clear, even though I have battled pimples most of my life, I am full of energy, and feel great. My kids are healthier since we made this diet a lifestyle and I will never go back to the way life was before.

When I got pregnant with my fifth baby I was more determined than ever to follow diet. I stuck to eating healthy morning, noon and night. Each morning I walked three miles and visualized the birth I wanted as I walked. I was determined to be as healthy as possible with this birth.

With this pregnancy I focused on working with my body. While walking I visualized taking oxygen to my uterus and my baby sliding down my birth canal in peace and love. As I was walking I would think about the baby crowning and how funny it would be if I burst out singing Johnny Cash's song Burning Ring of Fire. It always made me laugh at the thought of
singing that song while pushing my sweet little baby out.

Then on September 15 around 9 P.M. I was having light cramping. I told my husband that I wanted to go to Donna's house and get checked because the last baby had come so fast and she lives 35 minutes away. Once at Donna's she timed cramping and was convinced that it was braxton hicks. As soon as I went to bed that night all cramping stopped.

The next morning, an hour after waking up, I started having light cramping again. It was still a lot lighter than period cramps. Donna had two appointments in Vernal that day and she said she would feel better if I went with her just in case. So I went along for the ride. During the day I continued to have light cramps but nothing real. As each one was happening I said 'thank you' and told my body to open, open, open. As soon as her appointments were done I called my husband and told him that it was false labor and I would be home soon. As we headed back to home I noticed that the cramps where lasting longer. They were not getting stronger. As soon as we got back I told Donna that I was sorry for taking up all her time and that I truly felt like my body was not making any progress.

Donna handed me a cup of pineapple juice . While I was drinking the pineapple juice I had a cramp that was stronger. I told her "wow this one has a bite" just as the words were leaving my mouth I felt a pop and water leaking down my leg. I said "I think my water just broke" so she took me to the birth room and checked me. I was blown away when she said "You are eight centimeters dilated." I could not believe my ears and I asked her how can that be I am not even in labor.

Donna then started running around very fast getting all the birth supplies ready. I thought it was funny that she was moving so fast. I am not even in labor what's the big hurry? I still felt like birth was hours away. Just then I had a contraction and I felt like I had to go number 2 really bad. I ran to the bathroom. She ran after me telling me not to push. I was still thinking she was crazy I just had to go to the bathroom. I kept thinking that she was going to have a mess on her hands denying me bathroom rights. My next four contractions were five minutes apart and they were strong enough that I started focusing. I walked around the room telling my body to open, open, open. I thought about my baby sliding down the birth canal in peace and love. On the fourth contraction I got down into a squat and felt the baby crowning. I started singing without thinking about it. I was so surprised when I caught myself singing while my baby was crowning. Then as she slowly slipped out I gave one push for each of my family members starting with my wonderful husband. And once I reached my youngest child's name my little angle, Mercedes, came into the world. I turned around and sat on a sterile pad on the floor and held my baby while Donna suctioned out her nose and mouth. I was completely at peace and surprised that I was holding my baby when only 30 minutes before I wasn't even in labor. Mercedes never cried when she was born but she opened her eyes and when she was three minutes old started smiling. None of my other babies smiled that early. I truly believe that she felt the love I had for her and I had not forced her out but rather released her and she felt completely at peace with her birth as well. She weighted 6 pounds 9 oz and was 19 inches long. I have never felt such love for a baby. I truly believe that self hypnosis and Donna's wonderful diet helped me to give birth the way it was meant to be. To let our bodies do what they know how to do and completely surrender and let our babies come out into the world in peace and love.

~14~
THIRD TRIMESTER
Most common challenges and solutions

Braxton Hicks Contractions during the last four weeks Braxton Hicks Contractions are a sign of increased estrogen production in preparation of labor. Without adequate estrogen in the system the body can't start or follow through with labor. Braxton Hicks contractions are a sign that the body is preparing for labor and delivery. They should be viewed as a good thing during the last month prior to the estimated due date.
Possible Solution: A few drops of a lobelia extract in an alcohol base can be rubbed into the contracting area to help relax the muscles, without interfering with any hormone balance. A cup of Chamomile tea may also help to relax the muscles. These can be used as frequently as necessary to assist with comfort.

Braxton Hicks prior to the Last Month: shows potential for an early delivery and should be attended to.
Possible Solution: Sarsaparilla root tea or capsule form or a progesterone cream can add progesterone to assist in relaxing the uterus. It is advised that open communication be held with your healthcare provider if progesterone cream is used because some are strong enough to keep the body from going into labor and should not be used after 36 weeks for this reason. Once stopped it can take two to three weeks for the levels to drop enough for labor to set in if the cream has been used for an extended period of time. A good progesterone cream will have at least 500mg per ounce of progesterone.

Lack of Braxton Hicks Contractions: The absence of Braxton Hicks contractions, during the last month of pregnancy, is a sign that the estrogen is not increasing and the labor and delivery could be delayed, sometimes for two to three weeks after the due date
and is a primary reason for ladies going overdue.
Possible Solution: If you have not had any signs of Braxton Hicks contractions by the 37th week, one pint of soy milk per day or one black cohosh capsule two times per day can be used to start Braxton Hicks contractions by increasing the estrogen production. All forms of progesterone should be stopped.

Breech Baby Breech position is when baby is laying with head up, towards the ribcage of mom, and the little bottom down next to the pubic bone. Babies are far easier to deliver vaginally, if they are in a vertex (head down) position. If there is a lot of flutter movement in the lower abdomen then this is usually a sign of a breech baby. Another sign of a breech baby is if the heart tone is heard in the upper part of the uterus, above the naval. (*See the prenatal care section for more information on locating the heart position*). Breech position of baby can happen for few different reasons.

1) Not Enough Time Spent on Her Hands and Knees: Decades ago women spent more time on their hands and knees cleaning, gardening etc. These days women tend to do these things from a standing position or else hire them done.
Possible Solution: Pelvic rock exercises, described in the exercise section, should be done on a regular basis, from the first trimester on, so if baby moves out of place the chances are much higher of returning to the proper position. If baby is found to be out of proper position then do the exercises frequently, every 30-45 minutes for one waking day. Along with the exercises, Pulsatilla 6X is a homeopathic that has been applauded for many years for helping baby turn without tying up in the cord. Be sure to do the exercises twice per day for the remainder of the pregnancy.

2) Baby's Brain Lacks Volume Density: This happens more frequently in natural blondes than those with darker skin or complexion but can happen with people of all genetic types.
Possible Solution: Two tablespoons of Granulated Soy Lecithin can be added to the supplements twice per day. Lecithin oil or soft gels do not work for this purpose. Lecithin granules are high in choline and inositol, which has been found to increase brain volume density and assists the head being heavy enough to maintain proper position. Babies that have lecithin during their time in the womb tend to be highly intelligent babies which, is a very pleasant side effect!

False Labor is a sign that the body is trying to go into labor. I prefer to think of it as a trial run or preparing for actual labor.
1) Muscles Tightening: and causing discomfort during preparation of actual labor.
Possible Solutions: A little lobelia (liquid on an alcohol base) rubbed across the bottom of the tummy and a warm bath will help ease the contractions. True labor usually is defined by contractions that have a regular pattern and they do not stop with the lobelia or a warm bath.

2)Cramping: with or without nausea. A posterior cervix can also cause cramping similar to a contraction, but usually feels different from false labor. False labor will usually start and stop with the cramps being irregular and having breaks in between. Cramps from a posterior cervix usually remain steady without breaks and can be felt either across the bottom of the belly or else in the back. Nausea can sometimes accompany these pains. (*More about 'posterior cervix' later in this section*)
Possible Solution: Talk to your care provider about the possibility of adjusting the cervix back to its proper position. If this is the case, pain is usually relieved within a few minutes.

Fear can stem from worrying about the birth process or what is going to happen after the baby is born, such as "Am I going to be a good parent?" "Will I be able to provide?" There are many things that may bring worries or fears to an expectant mother. It is one thing to have concerns and be able to act on them for resolution. It is another to have emotion that instills fear that controls, or interferes with, life.
1) Over reaction: either introverting (pulling within) or extroverting (taking it out on others) are equally concerning and cause problems in their own right.
Possible Solution: Taking an amino acid called GABA which is available in 750 mg doses at most health food stores and is often used to stop over-reaction. A cup of Chamomile tea can be used to relax the mind. If the fear is paralleled with a rapid heartbeat then a liquid calcium supplement may be helpful.

2) Past Trauma or Impressions that makes one afraid to move forward emotionally.
Possible Solution: I have recommended a homeopathic called Rescue Remedy, which can be found at many health food stores or online, because it has been used for many decades for emotional support. Years ago a midwife explained to me the benefits of this remedy while I was in labor by saying, "It makes you feel like you are wrapped in Mother's arms". She was right, I felt very calmed by taking it during labor as it helped at both the physical and emotional levels. My husband said he also found success by using it when he was concerned about my well being when I was in labor. We were both happy with the results.

Caution: St. John's Wort is a common herb used for stress and fear but should be avoided during pregnancy as it works with the hypothalamus and can cause uterine contractions. St. John's Wort can be used during labor or after the birth of baby, but not before. St. John's Wort should not be used during the warmer seasons or climates as it can cause sensitivity to heat such as sunlight, warm baths, warm rooms etc. St John's Wort also should not be used by anyone who is on a prescription MAO inhibitor.

Floating Baby is when baby is staying high in the uterus and is not settling down onto the cervix. During that last couple of weeks the baby's head needs to make solid contact with the cervix in order to assist with cervical dilation and effacement. Staying high in the uterus prevents that needed contact.

1) Cord Wrapped: around baby and has baby tied in a position that baby cannot slide down to reach the cervix. This can be around the neck or any other body part.

Possible Solution: Do not attempt to manually move baby. Pulling on baby when you cannot see the cord is a bad plan. Taking Pulsatilla 6X with each set of exercises and doing the pelvic rock exercises every hour throughout each day may help. The Pulsatilla works with the electrical energy constituent, as opposed to the chemical constituent, therefore works with the energy to readjust the baby and cord properly.

2) Lack of Estrogen: needed to give the uterus integrity to hold baby down into place. This usually goes along with lack of Braxton-Hicks and this pregnancy can go a week or two over due because the uterus does not have enough strength. This is more common with women using progesterone or those who have had several pregnancies close together or in older
women who have had several pregnancies.

Possible Solution: After the beginning of week 37 a woman can drink one pint per day of Soy milk and / or one capsule of black cohosh two times per day to increase estrogen levels.

3) Lack of Brain Volume Density: prevents the head from being heavy enough to keep baby in vertex position. Baby is floating in water and gravity plays a major role. It is far easier for baby to stay in the right position if the head is heavier than the bottom. The bottom gets heavier if the mother has been consuming flour products.

Possible solution: Take two tablespoons of granulated lecithin twice daily to increase brain volume density. Also, stop all flour and potato products.

4) Too Much Time Sitting: When a woman is sitting for an extended time then baby is going to move so mother is not sitting on his head. Also, too much time sitting keeps baby
confined into a smaller space and does not allow for readjustment.

Possible Solution: Take time to go for a walk in the afternoon or evening. Stretching out and walking can allow the baby to settle down further into the floor of the uterus rather than being forced up from sitting. After a walk, doing squats for about five minutes helps to put baby down closer to the cervix. (*See how to do Squats in the Exercises Chapter*) This not only makes baby more comfortable but mother will find it easier to take a deep breath if baby is not pushed up into her lungs.

Insomnia is the inability to fall asleep at night, sleep walking, or the inability to sleep for a full night's rest.

1) Daytime / Life Stresses: that consume our thoughts and end up going to bed with us at
night keeping the mind going with repetitious, unwanted thoughts.

Possible Solutions: a cup of Chamomile tea before bed is a wonderful relaxant and is usually not strong enough to leave one feeling groggy the next day like valerian can do. A dropper full of the Bach Flower, White Chestnut, has been used, historically, for clearing the mind of unwanted or repetitious thoughts and has a good reputation with our ladies. Note: Melatonin is often used for insomnia but should never be used by anyone under 25 years of age, therefore should never be used during pregnancy.

2) Calcium deficiency: can cause the heart to beat too fast to allow one to fall into a restful sleep. It can also present with muscle cramps, pain or bruising.

Possible Solution: Taking calcium, a high quality brand not from a rock base, before bed should slow the heart rate and allow relaxation. A brand with several types of calcium in a liquid form is usually effective. Two tablespoons before bed is usually adequate. It is important to remember that calcium is quickly assimilated in your body and should slow the heart rate within 15-30 minutes. Calcium can be used with chamomile and / or white chestnut as they all work well together.

Muscle Cramps or Charlie Horses happen when a muscle, generally in the leg, will involuntarily tighten up to a point of causing pain and is frequently brought on with stretching. The instant reflex is to grab the muscle and rub it. This is an acceptable symptom reliever but it does nothing to resolve the base cause.
1) Calcium/Magnesium deficiency: will present in the form of muscle cramps.
Possible Solution: Take a liquid calcium supplement three times daily, taking one tablespoon in the morning, one tablespoon in the afternoon, and two tablespoons before bed. Most quality calcium supplements are balanced with magnesium and Vitamin D. Symptomatic relief should be seen within a few days then amounts should be reduced.

2) Magnesium/Phosphate deficiency: usually shows as a muscle cramp that is relieved with heat or warmth and worsened with cold and happens any time day or night.
Possible Solution: Cell salt #8 mag. phos. can be found at most supplement stores or online. Try a dose as directed on the label before bed and as needed throughout the day.

Low Back Pain This is usually seen during the last days or weeks of the pregnancy as baby attempts to slide down into the cervix preparing for birth. The muscles are trying to hold integrity and are stretching in a way that they are not used to. One of the first indications there is a problem in this area is the woman will subconsciously reach back and put her hands on her low back and then arch back. This is an attempt to get comfortable and relieve the pressure from the low back and hip area.
Possible Solutions: A warm bath to relax the muscles and mentally or sometimes even verbally giving the lower back muscles permission to move outward allowing the hips to separate, slightly, and allow baby to slide down without resistance.

Have a second party, usually the mate or family member, relax the muscles with a gentle massage that allows for the muscles to relax outward. This can be done by having the mother-to-be lay on her side facing the person working on her with her back down to the lower hip exposed. With olive oil or lotion, start at the spine about waistline level and gently pull the muscle directly outward toward her side (in a hand over hand motion). Repeat every couple of inches down to the upper thigh. Repeat this process four or five times. When finished with the one side, change positions so the other side can be massaged in the same manner. Most women will immediately comment on the pressure being relieved. This massage cannot be done by ones self, it takes a second person to reach and relax these muscles. This is a very gentle massage as opposed to a deep tissue type of massage.

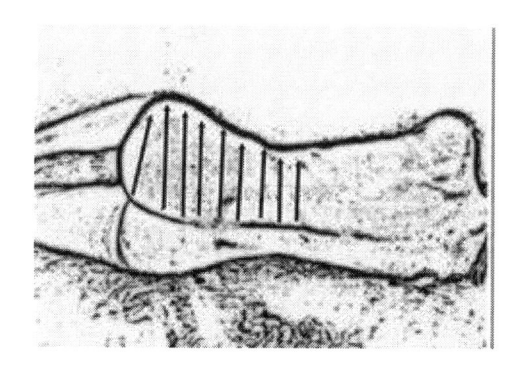

Premature Labor is when the body goes into labor earlier than is safe for the baby to be born. Anytime before 36 weeks is premature or baby being under 5 pounds.

1) Infection: will generally show up in a urine test as leukocytes and nitrites and by catching this early one could avoid premature labor. If the problem goes unnoticed then contacting the health care provider should be done immediately. To support yourself until you can get into the provider the following is suggested.

Possible Solutions: Taking doses of high potency colloidal silver 500 to 1100 ppm (every waking hour for the first 24 hours then cut back) and goldenseal root two capsules every four hours can help with the infection. Taking calcium and sarsaparilla could slow or stop the labor. Lying down (not sitting as sitting keeps the weight of the uterus and baby on the cervix forcing dilation and effacement) and remaining calm can help to stop any progression of labor until your healthcare provider can be reached.

2) Lack of Proper Nutrition: can bring on premature labor because the growing baby has nutritional needs and if they are not being met then the body may elect baby being safer outside the body with nursing.

Possible Solutions: Follow diet, eat the things that are good for you and leave out the things that are not good for you. Consume extra protein like that found in meat and gelatin. Gelatin has proven to be good source of protein that is easily assimilated. Drink the prenatal tea with red raspberry leaves, which are specifically used for strengthening the uterus and cervix. Most drink four to six strong cups per day. The tea should never be microwaved.

3) Hypothyroidism: (under-active thyroid) is commonly the culprit for premature labor. The thyroid hormones play a primary role in pregnancy and labor.

Possible Solutions: Taking a clean source of kelp increases the minerals that the thyroid needs for proper function. Any thyroid issues that have elevated during pregnancy may need more than just herbal remedies. According to my experience they require either raw glandular, homeopathic, or pharmaceutical support. I am not fond of using homeopathics for this purpose as they tend to be a symptom reliever, and if used should be backed up with a raw glandular. I have gotten the best results with a raw glandular that has 100mg thyroid with natural calcium, iodine, zinc, copper and l-tyrosine in it. Usual amounts are two tablets in the morning and one tablet in the afternoon. Taken too late in the day can cause insomnia. If the more natural remedies are not helping then medical attention should be sought after to help find a solution.

Sciatica is pain that can appear anywhere along the sciatic nerve which starts at the spine near the waist and down through the hip joint, then continues down through the leg making this the longest nerve in the body. The most common place for sciatic pain is in the hip.

1) Weakened Kidneys: are usually the cause of sciatic pain because the kidneys directly affect all of the nerves from the waist downward to the legs and feet.

Possible Solution: Stop drinking, or eating anything that would negatively affect the kidneys such as carbonation, sugar and high acid foods or drinks. Heat producers, like spicy foods can add to inflammation and should not be eaten. Any herbal diuretic with a combination of juniper, uva ursi, dandelion root and catnip to give support to the urinary tract.

2) Damage to the Nerve: (pinched nerve) will generally express itself by having pain that starts in one place and then generate to another area. Like, in the hip and then running down the leg or the pain consuming a larger area like the entire hip or low back.

Possible Solution: Three skullcap capsules three times per day to assist in the nutritional support of the physical nerve. Skullcap (also can be spelled Scullcap) has been used for centuries to rebuild physical nerve damage but is not used for emotional nerves.

3) Pain Not Relieved: by any of the previous measures may be helped by chiropractic or massage therapy as the adjustment of the tissue assists in the relief of many types of pain.
Possible Solution: Chiropractic or massage therapy, as long as they do not work on the uterus. There are several companies that put out a sciatic homeopathic and most are good for symptomatic relief and can be found at most health stores or online. If a homeopathic is used then the source of the problem still needs to be recognized and taken care of with either massage, chiropractics, nutritional support and/or change of diet.

Slipped or Posterior Cervix can cause a constant ache or cramp along the bottom of the belly above the pubic bone, and can usually be felt during the last couple weeks of pregnancy. Everything inside the body is held into place by an internal muscle. If there is not adequate protein and minerals then the muscle gets weak and allows the corresponding tissues and organs to slip put of place. The cervix is no exception. The cervix most frequently falls posterior (back towards the tailbone) when a woman leans forward or lays on her back while sleeping. However, if she tends to sleep on her right side, then the cervix will be found slid more to the right side, etc. Proper position for the cervix is when a woman is lying on her back and the care provider reaches straight inside the vagina and directly to the far end is where the cervix is to be located. If there is lack of proper nutrition, then the cervix can drop (become out of place) and instead of the cervix being found over the top of the baby's fontanel, the cervix is found down closer to the baby's nose (assuming baby is lying in proper position with head down and facing mom's back). When baby settles down into the cervix area the top of the head is going to miss the cervix and apply pressure on the low uterine wall causing discomfort to the mother. This is usually not off-and-on in rhythm but is more steady or constant and can be accompanied with a backache or nausea.
Possible Solutions: The cervix can be moved back into position as easily as it slips out by a health care professional inserting a clean, gloved finger into the vagina, inserting a finger into the cervix and moving it back to it's proper place. By holding the cervix in place for a couple of minutes or as soon as a pulsation is felt, and having the woman then slide into a squatting position for a few minutes. The cervix will most generally stay in place, alleviating cramping and nausea. However, if there is not an ample amount of protein or minerals in the body, the cervix is prone to slide back out of place again and the cramping and nausea will return.

I usually recommend one ounce of colloidal minerals (liquid minerals that have not been flavored or diluted) and two tablespoons of gelatin mixed into a warm fluid (chicken or vegetable broth works well). If a posterior cervix was a problem during any pregnancy, gelatin can be of great help if taken early during the following pregnancies.

Stretch Marks are caused from either growing too fast or from not having enough elasticity in the skin. The earliest sign of a stretch mark is usually a feeling of a deep itch caused by underlying muscles stretching to a point of tearing. If you find yourself scratching your belly, then start treating for stretch marks immediately.
Possible Solution: Watch diet remembering not to limit the amount of food you eat, just the kinds you eat. Sugars, breads, and carbonation tend to cause the skin to lose its elasticity and add to extra weight gain. Drinking plenty of healthy fluids and taking two capsules of evening primrose oil three times a day to replace the essential fatty acids has helped many. Rubbing olive oil into the areas of the breasts, hips and stomach that are prone to tear or wherever you are feeling itchy may help. By rubbing olive oil onto these areas each morning and evening one can usually avoid the dreadful marks that are so common. Once in a while we will find a woman who has existing stretch marks that are relieved by using olive oil regularly.

Notes

~~~~~A Short Story~~~~~

I delivered a baby for a couple that came to the United States from the Canary Islands. This couple had lived in several European countries, with a culture all their own, and were a very wholesome and health conscious couple. The night that she went into labor they had their own technique established. All the lights had been turned off and the only light that could be seen was from a closet door that had been cracked open and a few candles that had been strategically placed in each corner of their room. As I walked into the couple's room, she was quietly laboring on a blanket on the floor. As she approached transition, he sat on the floor with her head resting on his outstretched arm and with each intense contraction he would pull her up into his shoulder. He would then lean over and put his nose almost on her nose and they would gaze into each other's eyes through the contraction. Once the contraction was over, he would lay her back out at arm's length where they would both quietly rest until it was time for the next contraction. The tranquil mood never changed even through the delivery of their beautiful baby girl. Their parenting followed the same pattern of a peaceful and healthy lifestyle, as they were both hopelessly in love with their new daughter, they brought into the world. I will always feel blessed to have been their birth attendant.

~~~~~A Short Story~~~~~

The only woman I have ever witnessed giving birth without any pain was a beautiful Mexican woman. As she lay there cupping the face of her youngest child and talking gently to her, the top of this woman's uterus would rise up into a hard mound and she would quietly break away from her little girl long enough to look up at me, point to her tummy and say, "There is a contraction." She would then go back to focusing on her little one. I watched in amazement as she had about an hour's worth of contractions without any sign of discomfort. Finally, the baby began to crown, and I asked, "Do you feel a need to push?" This sweet woman turned and looked up at me, with a smile, and said, "Only, if you want me to." I replied, "No, by all means, do what is natural to you." As her baby started to present, I reached down to support her perineum and baby gently slid out. Once her baby was born and all necessary checks were made, this mother took her child in her arms and introduced the new little one to her older sister. This was truly, a perfect birth, a birth beyond even my expectations.

I arrived 12 hours later to recheck this mother and baby to find her and her six children dressed in white and she was up fixing dinner for them. I asked her how she was feeling and she replied, "I feel fine. Having a baby is not difficult or painful. We got our new child and we welcome her." Her husband was now gone to work and life was back to normal. It left me wondering if there was some kind of disconnect between body and brain and she was not able to sense pain at all. I asked her, "Do you feel pain when you shut your finger in a door?" She laughed and told me, "Oh yes, that hurts, but having a baby there is no pain." Later on she wrote me a note that read, "Gracias Donna por tu humanidad, dedicacion, confianza experiencia ... Irma y Max".

No Irma, Thank you, for a most beautiful experience! You are a treasure.

~~~~~A Short Story~~~~~

I got a call from a woman who was nearing her due date. She had been a school teacher and her personality was pleasant but very collected and business-like. She was never prone to over-react. She said "Donna, I am not sure why, but could you come out to my house? I would like to have you with me."

I inquired as to whether or not she was having pain, contractions, had her water broke? Anything?

"No, I would just like you with me."

I hung up and thought, "She is so calm, yet this is what a 'panic' is for her". I grabbed my birth supplies, jumped into the car and started towards her place, which was about 10 miles away on back country roads. I was hurrying because I sensed there was something major going on with her. Women who are progressing quickly will generally want their husband and birth attendant close to them, but unlike this woman they are usually showing other symptoms.

I got within three miles of her house and my cell phone rang again. It was her husband: "Donna, where are you?"

"Don't worry about that, tell me what's going on?"

"She is suddenly wanting to push."

"Where is she?"

"She is sitting on the toilet."

"Get her off the toilet, and have her get on her hands and knees on the floor." (This position takes the pressure off the cervix and allows more time before the birth than a sitting or squatting position would.)

He hung up the phone to help her onto the floor and was talking her into relaxing.

Minutes later, I ran through the door and up the stairs to their bedroom. I came around the corner and she was on her hands and knees, on the floor at the foot of the bed. I dropped my bags, scrubbed up and turned to find baby crowning. I knelt next to her just in time to guide her little girl into this world. Her total labor time had been about 10-12 minutes. Thank goodness she was in tune enough to call when she did.

~15~
TABITHA'S STORY

My Journey for more knowledge, passion about how my body works, and a better way of life began 10 years ago. I had severe digestive problems as long as I could remember and even once had a doctor tell me that I should be checked for crohn's disease.

After a couple of miscarriages, I found myself pregnant with twins and had an okay pregnancy, but soon learned that I would have to have a cesarean delivery because baby "A" was breech. I went in for a routine check-up on my birthday and found that I was seven centimeters dilated and had to rush to the hospital to prepare for surgery. Before I knew what hit me, my twins were born and I was left feeling sick, very depressed, and overwhelmed. After the twins' birth my digestive problems worsened, but I continued on through life and started walking and running like a mad woman to help with the depression. The depression left, but the digestive problems never did.

Fifteen months later I got pregnant with my beautiful daughter. I exercised and ran through this pregnancy and felt like this pregnancy was better. I planned on a VBAC and had very little knowledge of what to expect. Two weeks before my due date I started to feel nauseated and a little crampy. At my doctor appointment, I was checked for dilation and was four centimeters dilated with some very irregular contractions. My doctor must have had some big plans the next day because she stripped my membranes, and told me to get things ready and meet her at the hospital in a couple of hours. I went to the hospital like my doctor said, but the nurse was trying to send me home because my contractions were so irregular. Then the nurse said that I was dehydrated and so she gave me an IV with some fluids. Five minutes later my contractions started a pattern and were two minutes apart. My doctor came in to check me and found that I was seven centimeters dilated. My doctor then broke my water and started me on pitocin without permission. I was not allowed anything to eat or drink (not even ice chips) and was only allowed to lie on my left side to labor. I then made the biggest mistake by allowing an epidural. I felt so pressured and still to this day don't know why I did it because I don't feel my contractions. After the epidural I felt pain, but not contraction pain, but a severe pain in my middle back and the right side of my stomach that would not go away. I labored like this for eight hours before my husband and I felt that something was terribly wrong and asked for a cesarean section. When they went to give me a spinal block they found that the anesthesiologist had put the epidural in wrong and the catheter was almost completely out of my back. In the end I had a beautiful daughter, but a very long recovery. I remember waking up, in the hospital, gasping for air. I felt so close to death that it scared me. My blood pressure dipped down to 81/35 and remained this way for three days. I recovered, but fought depression and more digestive troubles.

My third pregnancy (fourth baby) came as a big surprise, but I felt healthy. I was running close to 30 miles a week and I really felt pretty good. I ran until I was 24 weeks along and was then told that I needed to stop. I went into labor two weeks before my due date and as usual went in for a check-up to find that I was seven centimeters dilated with no pain on my part. I didn't even think about a VBAC, as no one would ever consider it at this point, and I had my third cesarean section. Once again I was left with depression and digestive issues and combated the depression with running. This time I started running three weeks after my cesarean section because I could feel myself slipping into the darkness. After my fourth child we found out that my autistic son had a form of epilepsy called absence seizures (which looks like they are constantly day dreaming). We placed my son on a strict sugar free, gluten free, and casein free diet. I went on the diet for support and found myself feeling better than I had in years and decided that it was the gluten causing problems, so I stayed away from gluten from then on.

Tabitha

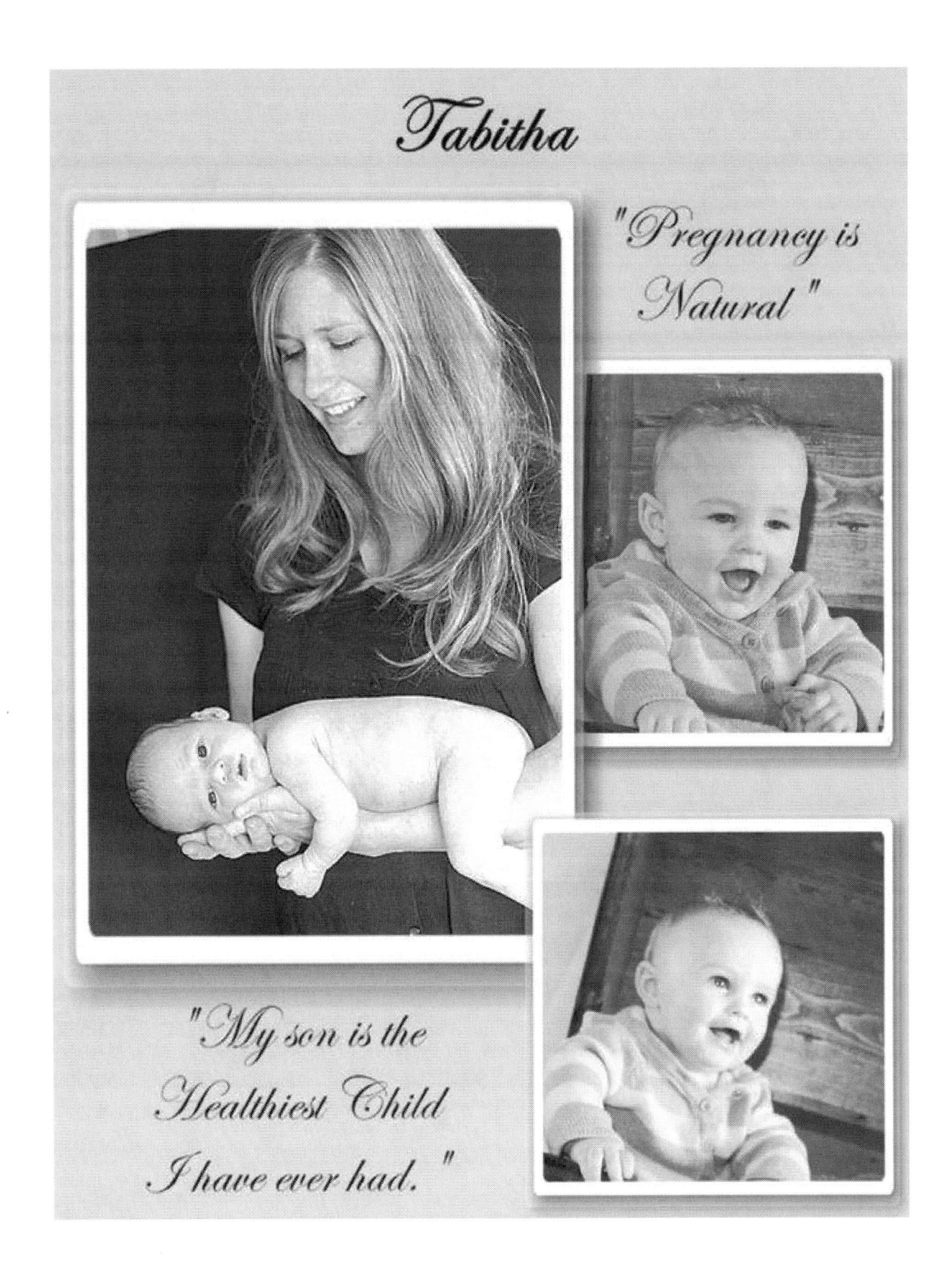

"Pregnancy is Natural"

"My son is the Healthiest Child I have ever had."

Almost three years later I became pregnant with my fifth child and immediately decided that I had to do something to avoid another meeting with death (a cesarean section). My friend Sherie had told me about her amazing midwife and the special diet that she placed her on. Her pregnancy was beautiful and the birth was amazing. She e-mailed Donna about me and asked if she was willing to try a VBAC after three cesarean sections. Well the rest as you probably have already guessed is history. Donna, who lived four and a half hours away was going to take me on as one of her girls and I would have all my checkups done by a girl that she had trained, that lived near by. I can honestly say that I followed ever ounce of instruction that was given, including diet. I wanted this more than anything and worked as hard as an Olympian. I walked three miles, five days a week and I had an amazing pregnancy. I had energy, my digestive problems went away, I slept like a baby my entire pregnancy, I didn't have the awful acne, and I felt amazing. I called her three weeks before my due date with some concerns. I was nauseated and started having that all too familiar crampy feeling (that wouldn't leave). She told me to start heading her way and was anxious for my arrival. We arrived at our friend's house and Donna soon followed. She checked my cervix and found that I was seven centimeters dilated and 95% effaced. Things were brought in and everything was prepared for a baby that wouldn't come. Yes, that's right. I was stuck at a seven for a few days and being extremely exhausted by this point, Donna stopped my labor. I continued to go in and out of labor for almost six weeks. I cannot even begin to describe the emotions and frustration my husband and I felt. At one point during this six-week period we gave up and went to a hospital for a cesarean delivery, but we were denied a c-section and sent home to have a VBAC. I still don't understand why I was denied, but I still laugh about a hospital denying me a cesarean delivery. No one knew why and no one had heard of such a crazy labor. I tried everything that I knew and I learned a lot about pregnancy in these six weeks, but it all ended in another cesarean section at a second hospital! This story however, does have a happy ending. Are you ready for the good part of this story? Well read on...

I had a beautiful baby boy whom weighed eight and a half pounds. My husband and I drew closer than we ever have before. I had a spinal block, but denied all painkillers except for the lowest dose possible of morphine added to the spinal block and I never had to have any other painkillers for 24 hours post surgery. I then had minimal doses of painkillers for only a few days after I left the hospital. They nicked a vein during my cesarean section, which caused a great loss in blood. My blood pressure still dropped very low, but Donna taught me how to combat low blood pressure and it worked. I left the hospital not even 48 hours later. My recovery was better than any I had in the past. I had adequate energy to take care of my family (I never had to have any naps) and there was no post partum depression to combat. I lost all of my pregnancy weight in the first week after the birth of my son. My son is the healthiest baby I have ever had he has had no hospital visits, no diaper rash, very little spitting up, and no colic.

The best part is that I have gained a very good friend out of this very crazy experience. Donna is on to something absolutely amazing and I can't wait to be a part of what she knows. I'm hoping to gain all the knowledge I can from Donna and I will, at some point in my life, become a midwife. I hope to educate women about their bodies and how absolutely in control they can be. I don't want another woman on my account to ever have to go through everything I have been through. There is a place for medicine, but pregnancy is not a disease or an illness that needs to be treated. Pregnancy is natural. I am grateful for modern medicine and its ability to help out in those rare cases, when things don't go as planned.

I still remain Donna's only girl that has followed directions and had a birth that ended in a cesarean section.

~16~
FATHER'S SECTION

Congratulations! Fatherhood is one of the most treasured positions you will ever hold. If you haven't caught hold of that vision yet, it is okay because it will happen when you get the chance to bond.

There is a lot that people, around an expectant mother, can do to make pregnancy a more blessed event, especially her mate. I will give some suggestions in this section that should help make your life a little easier and help you to understand what is happening. My goal in writing this section is to help give you solutions so that you are able to fit more comfortably into your role.

Everyone talks about how strange pregnant women are. They are really not so strange, but are beautiful and wonderful creatures that are listening to their instincts in a questionable world. I get along really well with most men because my interests are the same as his: we both want the safety and well being of his wife and their child. This is the way Nature works. You and your wife fell in love and as a result of that union a new little life is being brought into this world. She is responsible for protecting baby during pregnancy and you are responsible for protecting her. Over 90% of the time when you ask a couple, "If there had to be a choice made between mother and child, which would you choose?" The man will inevitably choose the mother and the mother will inevitably choose the child. A good husband is willing to give his life to protect his mate and a good mother is willing to give her life to protect her child. This is Nature's way of protecting both Mother and Child. This does not mean she loves the baby more than she loves you, it means she loves you as she always has and the baby is being brought into the equation. What has changed, is that all her instincts are telling her to protect the life within.

Unless circumstances alter the world, she is going to have a desire to secure things in her world for the new little one. This means getting rid of things that may harm, or not be good enough for the child. She may even go as far as dropping a hostile friend or not having as much to do with that friend until later. If there are things that are making her feel unsafe, then she will avoid it instead of confronting it, even if she would have done things differently before pregnancy. Her instincts will lead her to go where things are safe, instead of where they are fun. She will be more tenderhearted and will get her feelings hurt if she is not safe. If jokes are made toward her when she has the need to feel secure then it will be interpreted as being offensive. Your wife probably doesn't understand why she is feeling this way, but as you recognize that she is feeling this way, you will begin to see that it is because she is putting your child's safety first. Words do not secure safety, but actions do.

If our society did not take so much pride in girls with smooth abs, a nice slender figure, and unrealistic bodies then a pregnant woman would not have reason to wonder if her mate is still attracted to her ever growing and changing body. While young girls with hard bodies, are merely an illusion that the media has so creatively impressed into the minds of our society. This illusion leaves a lasting impression on women usually more than men. If she pulls away, give her gentle reassurance that you like the "new her" and allow your words and your actions to show her that you are changing with her and that all is well.

One day I observed a woman as her husband walked up beside her and patted her on the thigh. She brushed his hand away and said, "Stop that!" She had been accustomed to having a toned body and she was uncomfortable with the extra fluff that had come on with pregnancy. A few minutes later, he walked up and patted her thigh again, partly because he was teasing with her and yet, obviously there was something more. She turned around to him and lashed out, "I told you to stop it! Don't touch me there!" He looked hurt and backed away. I intervened and said, "Just a minute." While looking straight at him I said, "Do you like that?" He broke into a smile and said, "I do! I love the way it feels. It makes me feel close to her." She looked surprised and said, "You are kidding! I thought you were making fun of me being fat." He looked surprised at what she had just said. They talked about it for a minute and came to the conclusion that he did like her toned hard body, but in a totally different and loving way he was equally attracted to that little layer of softness that came with the pregnancy. It made him feel close to her and it made him want to protect her. Both were having changes they did not understand, but it was natural and from then on they were comfortable with each other because of their understanding of one another.

Sometimes a woman does not feel safe or may not be in a safe situation. She will think about what she needs to do to put the baby into the safest place possible. It can be her job, the neighbor, an insensitive mate, finances, or family that can make her act more offensive during pregnancy. She may instigate an issue to get people to move back and give her space. This behavior is telling those around that, "If you do not want to help in making this environment safe for my child, then you need to move back." If she does not have support from those around her, real or an illusion, then she will usually find a way to secure it for herself. If this does happen, it is the first step of moving back and it is a dangerous sign. It is a sign that she is not comfortable and Nature will have a hand in finding a safe place to have her baby.

There was a woman who had a strong willed personality, prior to pregnancy, and was quite aggressive and confrontational. If she got upset there was a tendency for physical expression. Her husband fell in love with her knowing what she was like and there was no attempt to change her. When she got pregnant, she changed and became very tender and loving. When she got upset she would walk into his waiting arms and bury her face into his shoulder and cry as he held her. He told me "I love this! It gives me the chance to take care of her and see her gentle side. I wish she could be like this all the time!" He loved his wife before she was pregnant, but he felt needed while she was pregnant.

Pregnancy obviously affects men differently than it does women. If you have solutions to her problems, other than useless advice, you become her hero. This book is intended to give solutions for the most common pregnancy concerns and if you don't find the issues concerning you in this section, please look through the rest of the book to find them. Here is a list of the most frequent concerns that fathers have.

"My wife complains, a lot" Understand that she is trying to figure out what is going on in her body. The good news is she can talk to you about it. She did not get a manual with her pregnancy and is trying to figure it out as she goes along. She was taught things, but she is now finding out that some of the things that she has learned don't go along with what she feels. She may begin to feel confused and even frustrated.

If she is talking about the same things over and over again, then the issue is probably not being resolved and you need to listen to what she is asking for. Whatever it is that is bothering her is more than likely, interfering with her feelings of security. Try to recognize the problem and assist with a resolution that she is comfortable with. Maybe ask her what she would like to see happen and then listen quietly as she tells you.

If it is a new thing each time she voices a concern, like an outside issue such as work or family, look for the common denominator. Listen to her and help her to find it and put the problem to rest. Is it always about work or responsibilities?

Take a look at her and ask yourself, "Does she look tired or is she pale? How many hours is she working? Is she taking time for her?" If she is working more than her body is comfortable with, her blood pressure can drop. When this happens every step she takes is an effort. By replacing the electrolytes, she should begin to have more strength and life will feel like it is less of a struggle. (*The electrolyte recipe is in the First Trimester section of this book*)

If the electrolytes are replaced and she is still pale, or if the inside of her bottom eyelid is pale, then she could be anemic. Try talking to her about getting a ferrous sulfate supplement, which is available at most pharmacies.

"She is always throwing up!" Yes, this is a common symptom with pregnancy. Most believe it is natural and some even believe it is a sign of a healthy pregnancy. Throwing up is not either of these and she hates it worse than you do, trust me. Support her with diet and eating things that are not going to induce nausea. If she is not feeling well, she does not have the strength to fix two meals each time (one for you and another for herself) so she is going to just eat what she thinks you want. Let her know that you are happy to eat the foods that don't make her sick. Help her plan meals that are healthy for her and filling for you. Read through the section on Morning Sickness in this book and see if you can help her find a solution. Help fix healthy meals for her and see if that doesn't help.

"She has weird food cravings" Those food cravings will usually form a pattern. If it is dairy, she is probably low in calcium or protein. If it is seafood she probably needs more minerals. If it is breads and carbohydrates she probably has low blood sugar, and her intake of protein needs to be increased. Look at what she is craving and try to find a connection. If she is craving everything, then it could be that she is worried, talking to her and allowing her to voice her concerns should help. Be gentle and she will more than likely open up. (*Read more on food cravings in the First Trimester section*)

"I hardly touch her breasts and she says it hurts" There are extra hormones produced during pregnancy and the hormone, estrogen, can sometimes cause breast soreness. This is more frequent if the sex of the baby is female, but can still happen with either sexes. The soreness is sometimes accompanied by enlargement of the breasts. You may think it looks nice, but it is terribly uncomfortable for her, even to the point of pain without being touched. Respect that it may be painful to have her breasts touched. Vitamin E is used to relieve breast soreness at doses of 400iu twice a day for a week then she can cut back down to 400iu once a day.

If the breast soreness is accompanied with uterine contractions then it can be a sign of a potential miscarriage. If there is enough estrogen to cause the uterus to contract then the pregnancy is being threatened. Do not touch her breasts, as this can make contractions stronger, and have her talk to her health care provider. I have my ladies take either three capsules of sarsaparilla three times a day (to stimulate Progesterone to counteract the estrogen) or I have them use a progesterone cream externally. The cream I use has 500mg progesterone per ounce. There is usually a change within an hour or so. I usually take them off the progesterone at the end of 13 weeks, because the estrogen threat is usually over at that time. If the breast soreness and / or cramping picks back up then I have them take it through the 37th week. After 37 weeks, we want estrogen so that her body can prepare for labor. Some deliver within days of stopping, others go to term.

"She does not like sex anymore" There are several reasons for this. The biggest one is usually fatigue, followed by being self conscious about her physical appearance. Read through the section on fatigue and try to get her to feeling stronger. She could be figuring it is normal, or she is just too tired to care. Once she is feeling stronger she is more apt to put out energy on something more than just trying to survive.

Next, she doesn't equate her new look to "sexy". Reassure her that she is beautiful and you would not change anything about her. Treat her that way all the time.

If there are cysts on her ovaries or a variety of other things, the pregnancy hormones can cause them to be more sensitive causing cramping with sex. This is uncomfortable and it triggers a thought in her mind that baby is being jeopardized. Find a different position that causes less cramping and be very gentle.

Her hormones have changed and she may be confused by the change. She may love just being held, without sex. If she does not get adequate physical contact between times of lovemaking, she may pull away during those times too. I have a close friend who has said "Men need sex to feel loved. Women need to feel loved to have sex." I think he is pretty close when it comes to expectant moms.

Sometimes a hormone imbalance can cause the vaginal muscles to tighten to a point of it being painful to be penetrated...the muscles would feel almost 'brittle' to her. This is not for lack of desire on her part, it just makes it painful because the muscles are not relaxing to accept her partner. In this case warmed olive oil can help. The olive oil is not only very healing but the warmth helps to relax the muscles. (You know cold constricts and warm relaxes? Yes, it works here too) Massaging her with warm olive oil prior to lovemaking can help. Be patient, it may take a few treatments to get the results you want.

Later on in the pregnancy pressure of having her belly pressed on is difficult for her, especially if it induces contractions. There is so much in there that her internal organs are pushed into different places to make room for the growing baby. Pressing on the belly causes added pressure to be applied to her lungs and heart and makes it difficult to breathe. It wrecks the mood if she cannot breathe. She, generally, wants emotional closeness and if you are behind her then the emotional part is lost. Hands and knees position is usually not a good plan for a pregnant women. The solution is usually to place her on her side with her shoulder tipped back so she can still see you and then be verbally affectionate during lovemaking. This relieves pressure from her, leaves emotional bonding intact and maintains satisfaction for both. Try different positions; be patient, gentle and loving.

Lovemaking is an important part of your relationship as well as being important to the pregnancy. Sex prepares the birth canal for an easier delivery. The hardest deliveries I have ever seen are with women who married as virgins and then had a difficult time with sex and only had sex six to eight times, total, before the birth. These births are very hard on mother and child because those muscles are not used to being used, therefore resist expanding for the birth. Resolving all the problems for sex and having a positive sex life during pregnancy is an advantage for all concerned. Be loving and patient in your day to day life, find resolution to the problems and both of you should be rewarded in a more positive physical relationship.

"She tosses and turns all night and I can't get any sleep" If she is tossing and turning, it is probably later in the pregnancy and she is having a hard time sleeping because she is uncomfortable. This usually happens during the last few weeks. Offer to fix her a cup of Chamomile tea sweetened with some Agave Nectar (Agave is sweet like honey without causing the glucose to rise like sugar and honey do. It also does not have the strong honey taste). Chamomile will usually assist in her powering down so she can rest better. A dose of high quality calcium could assist also. (Never give calcium from a rock base such as bone meal, oyster shell, coral etc. It will not break down to a cellular level to slow the heart rate for sleep.) A dose of calcium, or a cup of chamomile tea for yourself may also help so that any movement during the night does not disturb you.

"She has to urinate all the time" There are several reasons for this. One is her body's change in hormones. However, the biggest factor is that the fluid in the amniotic sac is changed several times a day, which means her kidneys must accommodate her needs plus the baby's needs and the amniotic fluid change. Be patient. It bothers her more than it does you. If it is because she has a weak bladder, then three capsules of the herb cornsilk can be used three times per day to strengthen the bladder. Sugar tends to weaken the bladder muscle and should be avoided. She could have sweets made with honey, agave, stevia or pure maple syrup that would not have the negative affect on the bladder. Carbonation is also hard on her urinary tract so having non-carbonated drinks for her would be a positive help.

"She is in her last month and she says her back hurts all the time" There is a battle between the low back and hip muscles and the baby, as the hips are trying to maintain integrity and strength, the baby is trying to move down into a position for birth. She will generally stand and place her hands on her low back while arching her back to relieve the pressure. A massage can help her with this low back and hip pain. The instructions for the massage you can do are found in the Third Trimester section in this book under 'Low Back Pain'. She cannot reach the muscles to do it for herself so she is relying on someone close to her, probably you. All you need to do is gently give those muscles permission to move outward and allow room for your child.

"She seems so sad." There could be several reasons for this. She could have problems that are not being resolved. Talk to her and see what she needs. Sometimes she can pinpoint the problem, other times she cannot. The most common problem comes from worrying about the needs of baby or another member of the household that needs to be taken care of. If the immediate family is taken care of, to her satisfaction, then it could be a number of other issues.

Sugar consumption plays a primary role in feeling a little sad, as most of the blood sugar in the body is stored in the brain for brain function. Too many processed sugars can cause an imbalance and can cause mood changes. If she can eat apples, bananas, grapes, even honey instead of processed sugars this can help to regulate her mood. Agave is my preferred choice of sweetener, because it usually does not interfere with the blood sugar or the energy levels and does not cause restless legs or sleepless nights.

If the problem is over-reaction then the amino acid GABA will generally stop her from over reacting and knock the edge off her emotions. When I try GABA on someone for the first time, I have the client think of a very sensitive issue. They will feel the emotion well up inside and it will generally show up in their expression. Then I have them dissolve the GABA 750mg under the tongue and we will talk about something else for about 15 minutes. At that time, I will have them think of the issue again that had them upset just minutes earlier. Usually they will smile and say something like "I can think of it, but the emotion is not so close to the surface, I am able to handle it now." Perfect, that is what we are looking for.

"Will sex help her go into labor?" Yes, sometimes it does. The hormones in the semen assists in the dilation and effacement of the cervix, during the times where the body is already trying to prepare for birth. For this reason sex is usually acceptable during any part of the pregnancy except 1) When she is having pain or discomfort or 2) When there are signs of a possible miscarriage such as cramping, any sign of blood, water leakage etc.

Many couples use this natural form of induction to try to bring on labor. If both sides are agreeable during the final couple of weeks then I have no problem with it. However, once labor begins or the waters have broken (with or without contractions) then it is absolutely forbidden due to potential infection risks to the baby.

"What is the deal with the birth attendant doing an internal exam on her?" This is a pretty touchy issue to a lot of people, men and women alike. Most women really want to avoid these exams if at all possible and most men are uncomfortable with another man touching his mate.

The reason for an internal exam (pelvic exam) in the early stages of pregnancy is to check for cysts, other abnormalities, and to check for pelvic width and depth to see if she has pelvic capacity to deliver a baby. In other words, to see if her pelvic structure is wide enough for a full term baby to pass through during birth.

The reason for the exam late in the pregnancy is to check for cervical dilation and effacement, as this usually tells how close to her EDD (estimated due date) she is. She should also have a softening of the vaginal muscle to allow for elasticity during the birth. Her cervix should be softening, thinning and beginning to open up a bit. Depending on how close she is to her due date.

I have had some husbands tell me they got angry because a doctor took the liberty of doing an exam on his mate without explaining what the purpose was. Others have told me they left the room while the exam was done to avoid a confrontation with the provider. Please do not do that. If you have questions, then ask them prior to the exam. Providers can get pretty "routine" and forget the human side to things, but that does not mean that the situation shouldn't be handled with tact.

I try to make it a policy of not doing an internal exam on a mother without her mate with her. She does not like this any more than you do and she would like to have your support during the exam. Just having your hand to hold and to be able to look at you softens the feelings of intrusion that go along with it. Secondly, if you get upset or angry then it makes it more difficult for her. She needs your support.

I remember when I had two babies within two years of each other and the doctor did an exam about every time he saw me. I got to noticing that every time I had an exam I cramped and spotted afterwards, but my husband could do almost the same thing, trying to check the cervix and seeing if something was wrong, it never hurt. Why? Because that is very sacred territory and only the mate should go there under most circumstances. It is not sexual on the part of the provider or the woman, but it is generally considered medicinal by him and intrusive by her. It is justified by medical explanation, but it can still feel intrusive.

I have never had a woman's mate get upset with me over an exam and I believe there are reasons for that. 1) I am always careful about keeping the communication open. 2) I explain the reason for the exam and ask for him to be present, if possible. 3) As the exam is being done, I explain to both of them what I am finding and what role it plays in the birth of their child. 4) I do not spend one second more in there than is absolutely necessary to get the information I need. 5) They are both given respect.

There was a Spanish speaking couple having their third child who needed to go to the hospital for an exam, because of symptoms she was having. The nurse came in, gloved up and got ready to do an exam on this mother-to-be. Neither one of them new very much English and as the nurse started to reach for this mother's pelvis, I saw an almost tone of panic come across our lady's face.

I asked the nurse to wait just a minute and then turned to the husband, called him by name and quietly said, "Would you hold her hand?" The husband, being accustomed to working with cattle, grabbed his wife by the hand and shoulder and threw his body weight into her to hold her down onto the hospital bed and said "okay, I got her!" The mother-to-be and the nurse both looked at me in shock. I shook my head and asked him to get off from her and then I took his hand and gently slid it into the hand of his sweet wife. Immediately I could see peace come across her face and she looked into his face while they gently held hands and the nurse did the exam. Then when the exam was over, the husband held their hands up together, looked at them, smiled and said, "Muy bien." (Very good) He found he had the power to keep her from having a bad experience.

"What is my job during labor and delivery?" You are her support person and her protector. During labor, different women have different needs and desires; some want their space while others want closeness. Some may talk a lot while other say nothing. While a woman is going through natural labor there's generally no bleeding, bruising, or obvious signs of damage. However, what she is experiencing is very intense and every woman has her own way of coping with it. Some women will want to walk through a contraction, while other's will walk between the contraction and stand still through the contraction. Some desire to be touched while others are distracted by touch. So the best thing to do is remember that it is her going through the intensity and you should follow her lead. If she wants you close, get close to her. If she is more comfortable with you out of her space, don't take offense by it just move back. This is just how she handles things. No matter what choices she makes, it is not a reflection on how she feels about you. Even if she prefers you to not be close, she will usually want you close enough to hear what she says without exhorting too much energy.

Encourage the atmosphere to be quiet and relaxing for her. Loud talking, subjects such as last week's football game, or the latest business transaction are usually unacceptable. Phone calls and the rest of the world can wait. If someone in the room starts to talk about an uncomfortable subject for her then you can have them hold that conversation somewhere else. This is her hour(s) and she deserves to have respect. Watching television while she is laboring is not a good idea unless she wants to watch something, leave it turned off and focus on her. Offer her ice chips (or whatever the birth attendant allows) and don't let her get dehydrated. If she is hot, a cool cloth will be appreciated. If she is cold then get her a blanket or something to warm her up.

Words of encouragement are always accepted, especially during that last part of labor. "You are doing wonderful" "You are doing this with such grace" "I am so proud of you" are all good words of encouragement.

I have had women that give their mate instructions such as, "If I start to push, remind me I want to just relax and let the baby birth at her own pace", or "I want to listen to music during labor" "I don't want a c-section so you see to it that they don't give me one." These are things she trusts her mate to enforce. Things need to be written down for you, along with the birth plan for the birth attendant. Get it in writing so you don't forget. If you get into the birth and she changes her mind or there is a safety issue involved then changing plans for the safety of your wife and baby is always the best plan. If in question about a medical emergency, if something is not quite right, then you are entitled to a second opinion unless it does not allow time. Be familiar with the causes for a c-section and an understanding of how the birth process works so that you can know when you are getting valid information.

Remember that while you are in the hospital there are patient rights and you can ask your hospital for a copy of theirs. Patient rights are for the protection of the patient and family as well as the hospital. They are generally fair and balanced for all concerned. (*A sample of Patient Rights is listed in the Labor and Delivery section)*

Preparations made ahead of time help things run more smoothly. Know enough about what is going on to recognize a natural process from a complication. Remember that she is vulnerable during this time and you are entrusted to be her protection and emotional support. You can do it. Remain calm, supportive and alert and everything will work out just fine.

"How long do we wait before having sex after the birth?" Women are all different and depending on how well the birth went, there are different degrees of damage that may have been done during the birth. If there were tears or an episiotomy then it will take longer than if it was a smooth, natural process where there was no damage to the birth canal, perineum, or cervix. If there was a tear, or episiotomy, then enough time needs to be given to allow those areas to heal. There is always the open site where the placenta was attached to the uterine wall, which needs time to heal. It is important to give her body a chance to heal properly before any kind of sexual activity is performed.

As long as there is bleeding then there is something that is not, yet, healed. Sexual activity can increase the chances of infection getting into the open wounds. Sex can also open up areas that are sutured. The sutures are there for a reason. There are muscles that go from the inside of her hips down to the pelvic floor (perineum) to hold her hips into place. Women who have tears (or episiotomies) that are not allowed to heal properly have a much higher chance of having long term low back and pelvic pain than other women, this would be a long term pain for a short term desire. Allow her pelvic floor to heal.

I approve clients to resume sexual activity as soon as 1) There has been no bleeding for 48 hours or more. 2) She feels up to it <u>and</u> there is no pain involved. 3) There is no odor of infection or any other discharge. When all of these are good then I give the go ahead; but never before that.

The first few times it is good to use warm olive oil, as a lubricant, to help heal and restore the natural elasticity to the muscles. It is also important to take it very slow and easy as to not cause any damage. If there is any pain, then stop immediately.

If you bump the cervix, (it will be very tender to her-like you are penetrating too deep), then it shows that the cervix has not healed yet and could be dropped down. It would be good to give it another week or so. If she could do some crunches, or situps, then it would help to pull that cervix back up to where it belongs and it will not interfere with sex. The best way to do this is to do as many as she can without pain and then stop, even if that is only one or two. Wait three or four days and, again, do as many as she can without pain. Generally, she can do two or three times as many setups the second time as she did at first because the time was given in between to heal those muscles from the initial exercise. Every part of the body is healed through diet and rest. It is torn down, in preparation to rebuild, with exercise and day to day life. So the pattern is to exercise one day then eat properly and rest (the respective area) in between exercise sessions and exercise again in three or four days. If bleeding increases during exercise then her body is not ready for it yet and it is causing damage.

Once the body has had a chance to heal then try again. Most of our ladies are able to resume an active sex life within two to four weeks after giving birth. However, rarely does one of our ladies have severe damage with her birth. Those conditions would be expected to take another two to four weeks to heal. By exercising patience, love and compassion your mate should be able to heal properly.

Notes

~17~
MANDE'S STORY
(By Donna Young--approved by Mande)

Mande had her previous three children in hospitals. Her birth experiences left her very unhappy. Her complaints ranged from insensitive birth attendants, forced procedures, inductions, and lack of control of her own births. She suffered from lack of nutritional support and needed counseling. She gained 30 to 50 pounds during her pregnancies and she was generally unhealthy. Her labors were longer than she wanted and difficult. Mande and her husband, Dean, knew there had to be a better way so they continued to search. Dean worked and went to school and Mande was a stay-at-home wife and mother.

Dean and Mande heard my contact information from another midwife when Mande was about 12 weeks pregnant with their fourth child. When they called to schedule their first appointment Mande was suffering from morning sickness and we discussed the causes of it and she went right to work to do her part in resolving the problem. By the time I saw her for the first appointment the problem was gone.

Dean and Mande drove over 100 miles to have their appointments. They were open to the changes expected in this program. They asked many questions and wanted things clarified so she could follow the program. Dean was supportive and eager for the change as they had already seen the changes in her health in the days prior with just one part of the program.

Over the next few months they would work together, as a team, to change their family's diet. Mande's health continued to improve and they started seeing improvements in their children's health as well. They were wonderful to work with. When they had a problem or questions they called, we talked about it and they did their part to resolve it. It always worked out well with resolution to the issues.

When it came time for their child to be born, I traveled to them. I arrived and within a few hours she was in labor. I was pleased to see the support that Dean gave his wife and the way she responded to him. Mande's mother was there and was also supportive of their efforts. Mande was in complete control of her labor and her vitals were good. She was up moving around and smiling with this beautiful smile between contractions. Her color was good and her body language showed she was at peace.

As a medical student and experienced father, Dean desired to deliver his own child and because this was a low risk pregnancy and birth I agreed to it. I would stand at his side and walk him through, teaching him proper technique as to not damage mother or child. It was an absolutely beautiful birth with little Wyatt being born into the hands of his Daddy. Mande's mother watched over and supported Mande and little Wyatt. Her total labor time was 90 minutes, from first pain to first cry. Dean and Mande were pleased with the outcome.

As circumstances would have it they moved 400 miles away. Mande went to school and became a Certified Doula and loved the interaction with other mothers. Though the births she attended were hospital births Mande enjoyed her work and continued to learn. Mande had time to decide what she wanted different with her next birth and, like some of our other ladies, Mande wanted to try to deliver her own child the next time she was pregnant. She knew it would require dedication and preparation and she was willing to put forth the effort to accomplish her desire.

Wyatt was born into His Daddy's Hands

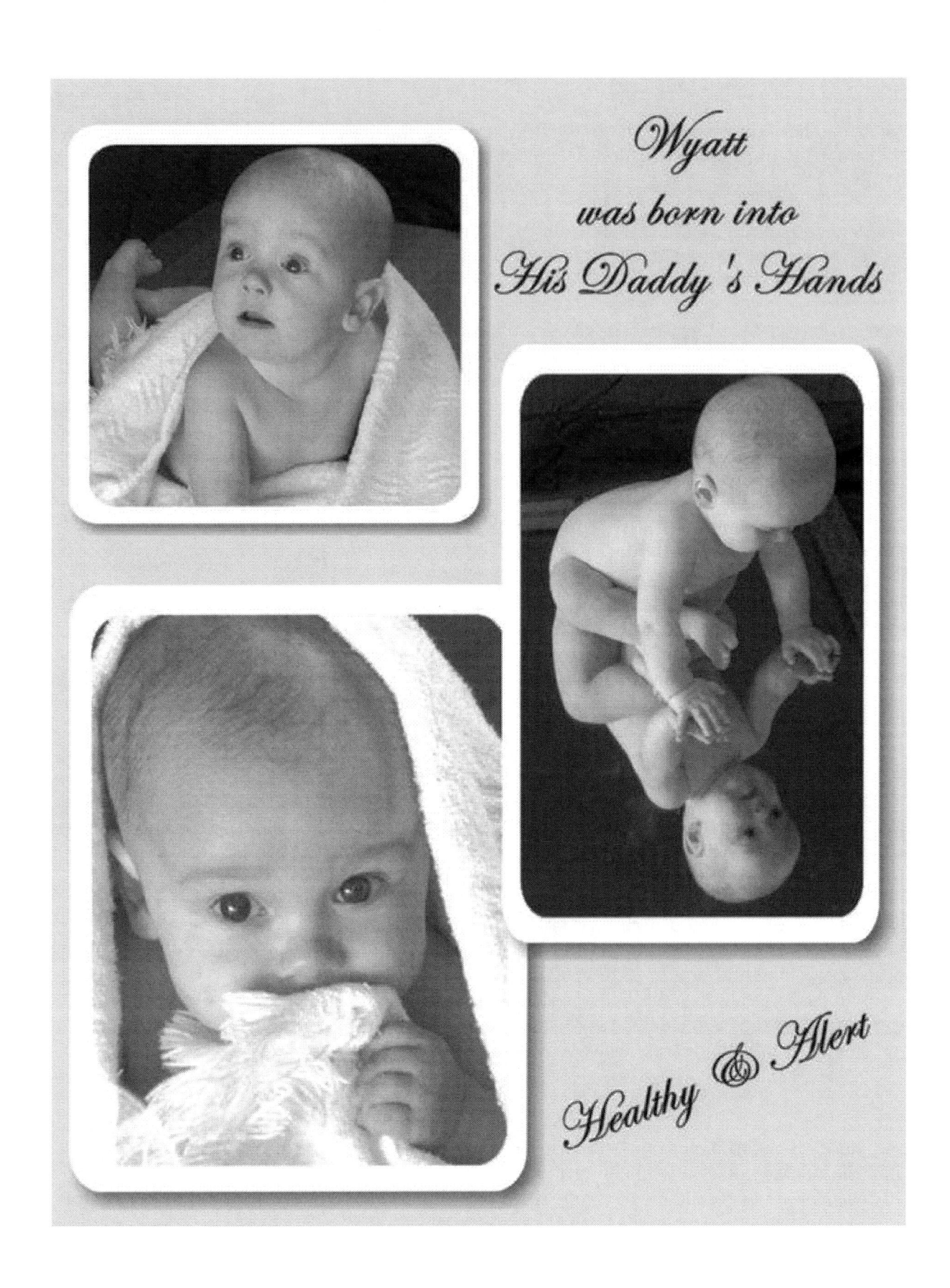

Healthy & Alert

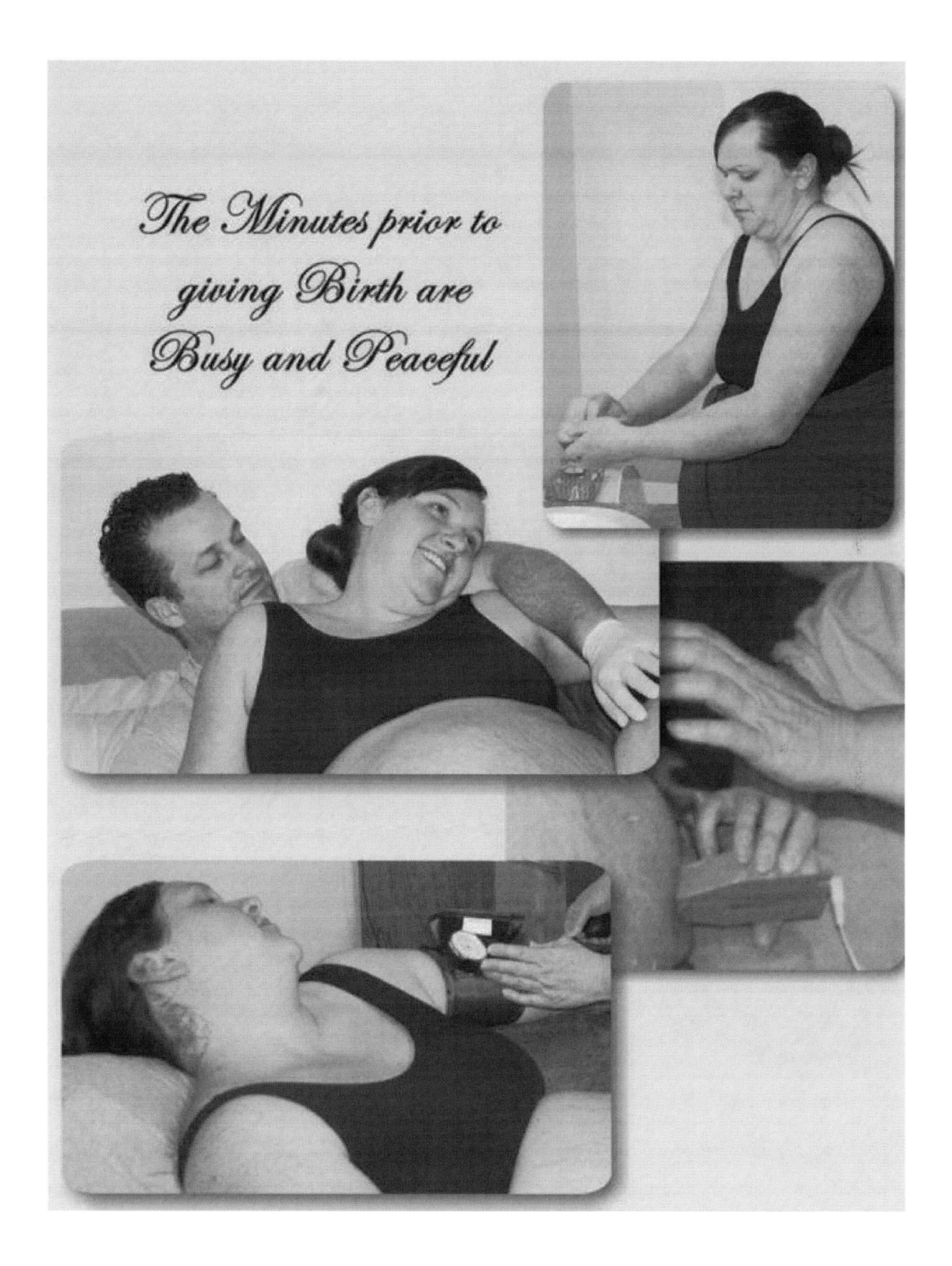

The Minutes prior to giving Birth are Busy and Peaceful

Jharyka's Birth

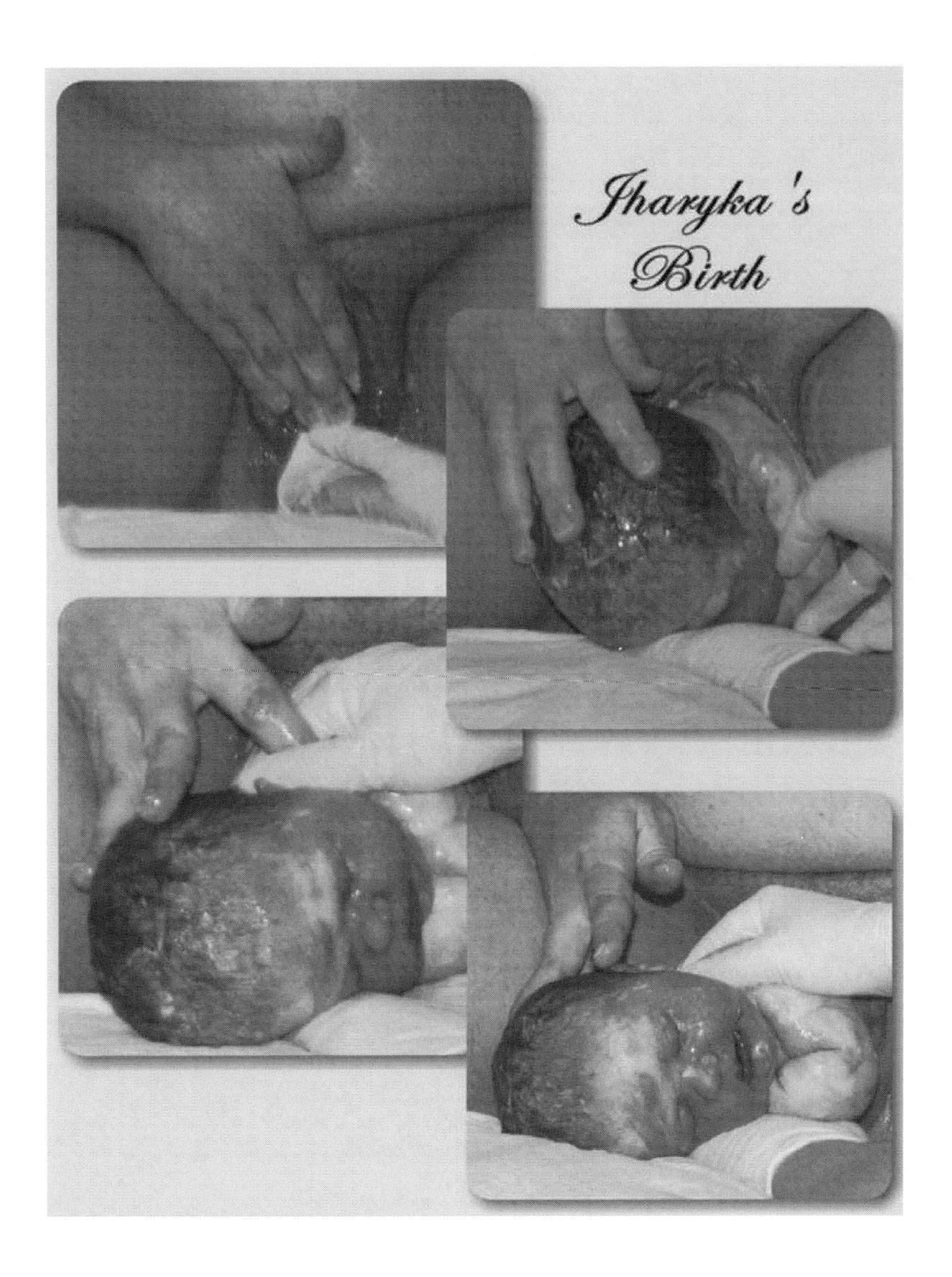

Immediately after the Birth

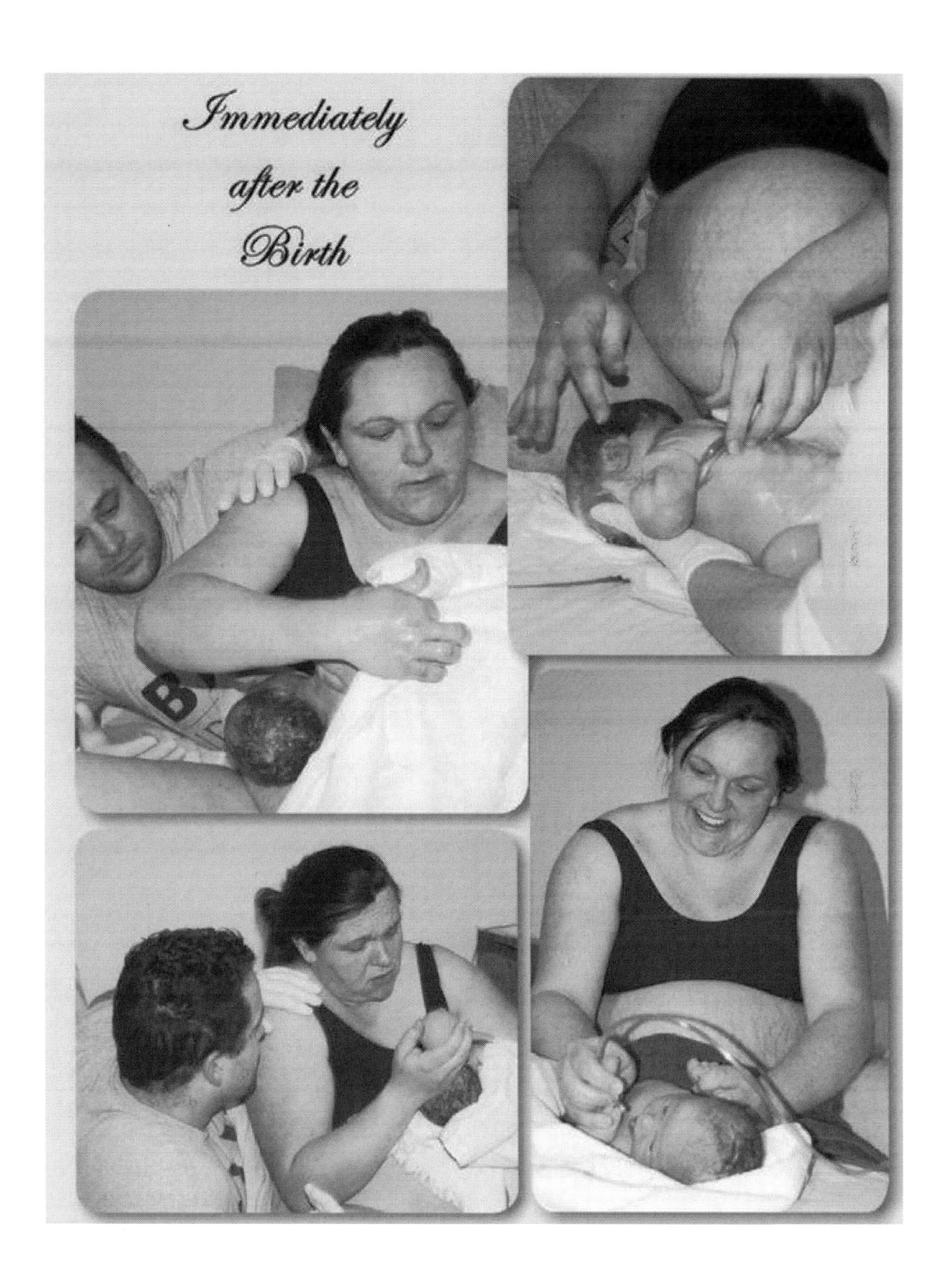

The Hour After

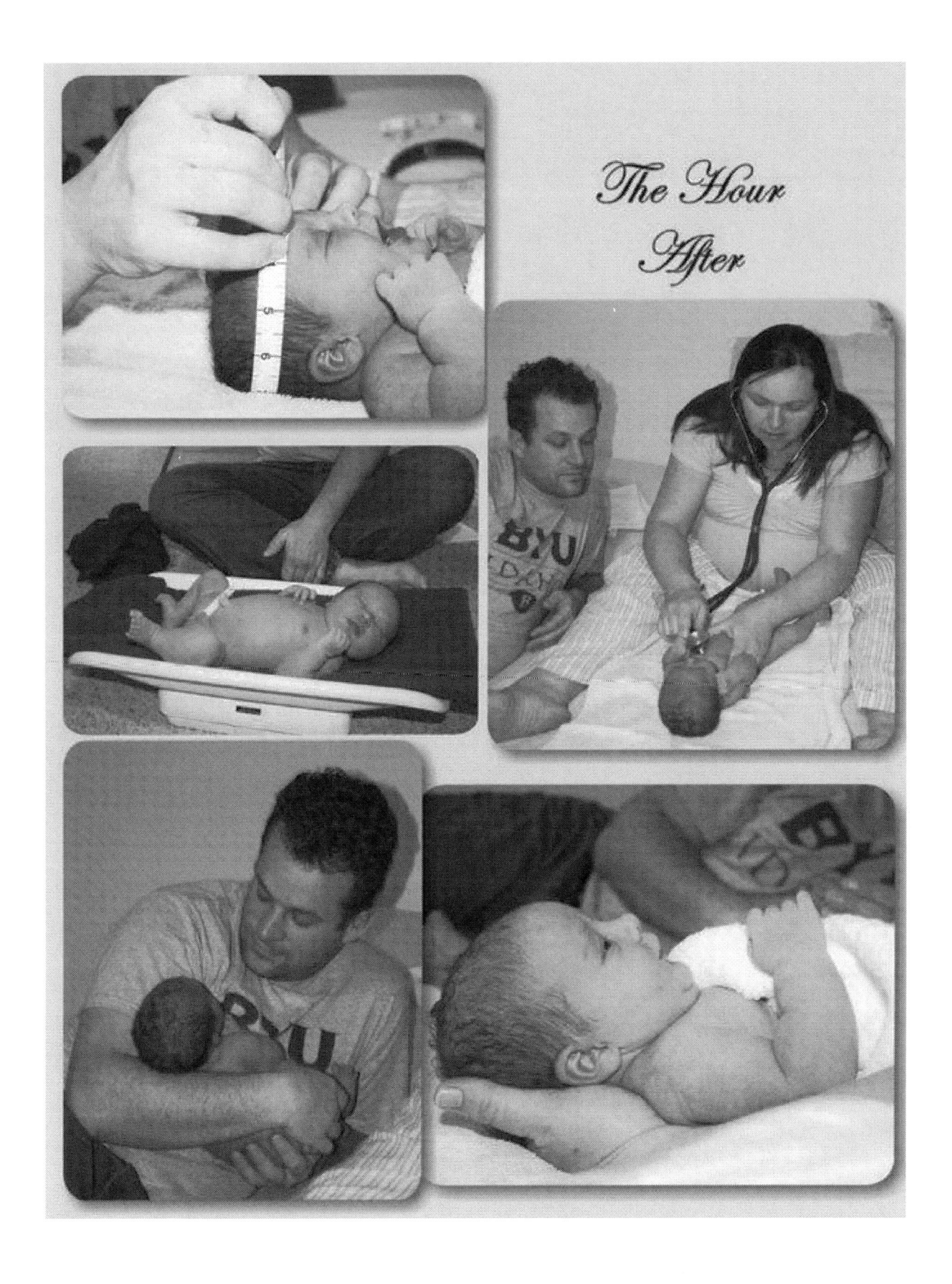

Mande got pregnant with little number five. She called and asked me to assist her in the birth of her child. They would come to my area and deliver locally at the home of a friend, who was also on the Powerfully Pregnant program.

Prenatal exams were done through Kala, a midwife who trained in this program for about five years, in Idaho. When issues arose we would talk it out over the phone. I saw Mande three times during her pregnancy and she saw Kala the rest of the time, followed up with a phone call with me to discuss results. Mande's pregnancy went well without complications.

With Dean and Mande staying in their friend's home for about two weeks prior to the birth, these couples had time to share recipes and ideas for improving their health. They were a wonderful support for each other.

On the night of the birth, Mande was again controlled and positive. Her vitals were checked regularly and were good, she had a focused state of mind. She was up moving around and cheerful and shortly before the birth Mande and Dean both scrubbed and he gloved up. Even though Mande decided she wanted him behind her for support he was ready in case she needed his assistance. She lay on the bed, which was the position she felt gave her the most control of her body and the baby. Minutes before the baby was born, Mande flashed a heart-warming smile in between contractions. The atmosphere was calm and this couple did wonderfully.

As Mande felt the baby's head starting to crown, she reached down to give support to prevent a tear. I gave rectal support. She gently pushed her baby toward her own hand. The contraction stopped and Mande took a moment to relax and breathe. Then on the next contraction, Mande gave a controlled push and eased her child's head out of the birth canal. Taking a moment for me to check for a cord, then Mande finished birthing her baby. Sweet little Jharyka took her first breath at 4:09 a.m. on February 26, 2010. Pictures reflect the peacefulness this beautiful child had during her birth and there was no blood on baby which says there was no tear on the mother.

Mande took the cord off Jharyka's chest and immediately took action to care for her own child. I handed her a sterile towel and she cleaned fluid from her baby's face, then reached for a bulb syringe to clear Jharyka's nose and throat. Jharyka then had a clear cry, but was slightly purple with an APGAR of 8. Mande gave her blow-by oxygen and Jharyka responded with a beautiful pink color and an APGAR of 10. Jharyka's eyes were bright and alert and she responded to both of her parents by turning to look at them when they spoke. She gazed intently into the eyes of her parents shortly after being born.

Dean stayed in the picture and assertively helped his wife care for their new daughter. Dean weighed Jharyka and helped check all of her vitals and measurements. They fulfilled their dream of taking full responsibility for the birth of their own child with a beautiful outcome. Mande is strong and capable of taking a lead role in caring for her child right from the moment of birth.

Forty-eight hours after the birth, this family left to return to Idaho. Mande and baby were checked and there was no reason for them to stay in Utah. Mother and child were both strong and healthy and ready to travel home in the capable care of Dean.

~18~
SINGLE MOTHERS

The information in this section actually applies to all mothers-to-be but it's especially important for the single mothers.

Single mothers can be categorized into two different groups. The first group consists of women whom, for whatever reason, find themselves outside of a committed relationship alone and pregnant. The second group consists of women whom are married or in a committed relationship and the father is gone working, in the military, outside of the country getting legal work completed, death of her mate, or some other issue that has them apart during the pregnancy or/and birth of the baby.

Single mothers not only have their pregnancy to focus on, but they are generally working outside the home and have to figure out a way to provide a safe environment for their child to be born into, away from physical or emotional threat. Pregnancy, in single moms, is something that is usually not planned and because they are left alone they have less time to adjust to their circumstances. The demands on a single mother, women in an unstable, or abusive relationship are greater, which causes a need for extra care.

For the Single Mother
Recognize that the child in your womb is not a mistake, a crisis, or a personal catastrophe. This is the most beautiful opportunity to bring someone into your life that will love you unconditionally. He/She will not judge you for any reason asking only that you provide love, food, and comfort. This child does not care how much money you make, your social or marital status, your political views, or what the neighbor thinks. Your child loves you and believes in you, just the way you are. You are your child's hero and no one else can take your place.

Your child loves you with the purest of love and is counting on you to feel wanted and loved. Your baby can feel every emotion you feel and needs you to be happy and feel secure. Your baby believes that you will do everything in your power to protect and provide the best health you possibly can. Know that you are 'needed' by your baby more than anyone will ever need you. What an honor and a privilege to have the care and trust of such a wonderfully innocent and vulnerable person placed in your arms.

Build a strong support system so you can focus on the extra work you have to do. Surrounding yourself with people who are supportive of your approach to your pregnancy and avoiding people who are judgmental or try to push their ideas or thoughts onto you is probably a good plan. No one has the right to ridicule your personal choices or convictions as long as you are making healthy and positive choices. Give yourself permission to do what you feel is right for you and your child. Make all your decisions with a pure heart and without shadows of selfishness.

I once knew a single mom who found herself in a position where other people, occasionally, took it upon themselves to voice negative thoughts (like they were telling her something she didn't already know or what they thought she should do). She was devoted to her child and to the safe boundaries she had already established in her own mind. One day someone volunteered a negative comment to her about her being a single mother and she looked the person straight in the eye I heard her say in a very calm tone, "Keep it nice or keep it to yourself. My personal life is exactly what it is: personal". The person stopped and said, "You are right". The subject was changed and all was well. People can only intrude as far as we let them and she stopped the intrusion on the first sentence.

If the pregnancy and birth are handled with proper care and support, this will be the beginning of a very close-knit relationship that can last a lifetime. At each prenatal appointment, you need to hear the growth and development of your child, not just cold clinical data. Pregnancy should be treated sacred and not as a disease or physical ailment, it is pregnancy--a new living child growing within. You need to feel empowered, to bring this child into your world, with beauty, grace, health, strength and dignity.

Who should I choose as a birth attendant or caregiver?
It's important to find a gentle, caring, and knowledgeable birth attendant that will give you the extra care and encouragement you need. The birth attendant needs to be able to answer all of your questions and put forth the extra effort to make you comfortable with your situation. It will be hard to feel at peace and to make good choices if you don't understand the changes occurring in your body or the process of birth. Knowledge will help you to feel empowered and help you to be actively involved.

Who should be with me during the birth of my child?
During your pregnancy, watch the people around you to see who is supportive of you and your approach and who is genuine. A person that carries the qualities you are looking for should be asked to be with you during labor and delivery. A person who you feel obligated to like a friend that will never speak to you again if she's not invited, an uninvited mother that is planning on being there, or any person who is pushy about attending the birth are not ideal people to have while in labor. This is a time when you need someone who is there for 'you' and will not be controlling. Baby and yourself should be the only obligation you have. It is better to be alone with a good birth attendant or healthcare provider than with someone who won't be of help to you.

The need to work harder and focus more than you ever have will be more difficult if there's a person who is causing you to feel stressed or distracted. Distractions make labor and delivery more difficult and can easily slow any progression in labor. Your support person needs to be exactly that, *your support* person.

What about making a birth plan?
Talk to your health care provider and tell them how you envision your delivery. Write down any desires you have for the birth and who your support person(s) will be. Making arrangements to hold baby immediately after the birth, will allow you the opportunity to have a better bonding experience and allows baby to look into your eyes, and put a face to the voice he/she has listened to for the past few months (Yes, babies can recognize familiar voices). This first eye contact is very important.

Holding baby immediately after the birth will allow you to examine every unique little feature of your baby. This may be more difficult to accomplish in a hospital environment, but as long as arrangements are made in advance and everyone is on the same page, things should go as planned. Just make sure it does not take too long before you get the chance to bond. The best time to bond with your baby is in that shining moment when adrenaline and energy are at their peak.

When I think back to a single mom who took the time and forethought to plan and prepare, my thoughts turn to a women who was a massage therapist. She came to me knowing she was going to be a single mother. She told me the situation and explained what she wanted and how she envisioned her birth experience. Her plans were reasonable and as time passed she worked out details that would support her own desires for a safe and peaceful birth. She was faithful in attending her prenatal appointments and doing her part for her child. She recognized that the choices she made each day played a role in how things would go in the future, for both of them. As the third trimester arrived she had all the 'who, how and why's' figured out. She had made all the arrangements and exercised personal responsibility.

As the birth neared she came to me with a plan of where she would have her baby and who would attend. She chose not to have her baby in her own home, because she wouldn't have anyone to help her after her baby was born. Her employer, who was also a chiropractor and her mentor, offered her own home for the birth. The mentor had room for her with privacy and all the things she needed. She chose her mentor and another person, who was an acupuncturist, because these were people she felt safe with. We talked about her support team and her reasons were based on significant forethought, and not from obligation, or pressure from any third party. Everything was planned with only the best interests for mother and child in mind.

On the day of the birth, I arrived and she already had her support people in place. I observed as she leaned on those she knew and trusted. She had chosen exactly the right people to be with her. Both of them focused on her and her comfort. No one crowded her, but they were there when she needed them. Topics of conversation were always within the comfort range of our mother-to-be. They offered ideas and she was open to their ideas, even though birthing was not their line of expertise. Her support team had everything she needed, and this had been recognized months earlier, giving everyone plenty of time to prepare. I allowed her the space to lean on her support team and also offered input, but I know that it is always the 'mother-to-be' that has to do the work. She delivered her child, her way, in her own time and did it with pure grace and dignity.

When her baby was born and the airways were clear, baby was given directly to this glowing mother. She tucked baby close to her heart and her beautiful little girl looked up and gazed into her mother's eyes. It was a sacred moment when the two of them caught eye contact for the first time. They were finally able to see each other and this was a truly magical moment. We stood there watching the honest and pure love these two had for each other. The two of them had just stepped into a new world and were beginning a new and beautiful journey together. They had each other and nothing else mattered.

This is a perfect example of a single mom stepping forward to give her child all the love and beauty her child deserves and needs. This woman has always held a special place in my heart for the devotion she still continues to have for her child. From the moment she knew she was pregnant, she did everything in her power to provide a positive environment for her child and she never let anyone make decisions for her. This single, working mother, has always put her child first.

For the Support Person
If the father is unable to attend the birth but they are still together as a couple, the mother will usually want to hear wonderful things about him. It's always nice to complement on how proud the father would be if he could see the wonderful job she is doing. After the birth of the baby, mother usually likes to hear the ways in which baby resembles the both of them. Including the father into the conversation is generally what she wants and needs unless she has negative feelings towards him. You, as the support person, should know whether or not the father should or should not be brought up in any conversation. Find these things out ahead of time.

If this mother who is truly alone, I have found it best never to mention the father because of the negativity that may be associated to the birth. It is best to allow the mother to have this beautiful time to herself, with the cares of the rest of the world left outside. The mother will usually choose the subjects that she feels comfortable talking about and if she should bring up worries or fears, it is best to give her positive reassurance that everything can be worked out later. Her focus should be placed on her and her baby.

Choices
Being a single mother requires more preparation, and you are fully capable of providing what is best for your child. Making choices with good intent, without selfishness, and acting on those choices will be a reflection of the devotion you have to your child. Make your choices well.

Video Taping the Birth
For the temporarily single mother, taping the birth may be even more important. The women who will not have their mate with them may want to tape the birth so that it can be shared. She may want to share the video with him upon his return or send it to him, or share with her family, or close friends. The ability to share this event with her mate as soon as possible will, generally, mean the world to both of them.

For single mothers who are completely alone, taping the birth can be a nice reflection on a beautiful memory. Single mothers don't have a mate to tell them what a wonderful job they did and having the ability to look back later, as an observer, is usually a positive experience. Note: A tripod, strategically placed, is a better plan than having the support person spread between two jobs. Let the support person just be support.

NOTES_____

_____

_____

_____

_____

_____

_____

_____

_____

_____

_____

_____

_____

_____

~19~
MELISSA'S LETTER

Hi Donna,

I just wanted to say hi and tell you I have been thinking about you lately. I had the opportunity to go and watch a friend give birth to her little boy on Monday, two days ago. So it has been on my mind a lot. She was induced and given an epidural. While we were waiting for her to dilate, the subject of me having had a natural home birth came up. The nurse said something about how she delivered her babies naturally. Then, my friend's husband (his wife was currently in labor with an epidural) said "why would you do that, what is the benefit, just that its less expensive?" Well, I got really nervous about expressing myself and answering the question and decided that it was not the time or place to bring up MY reasons for wanting a natural home birth. So I just kept quiet and the subject quickly changed...thankfully.

Well, her epidural inexplicably stopped working when she was dilated to an 8. I am sure you can only imagine, but she was suddenly hit with hard contractions, unprepared for the pain with no explanation. They called the epidural guy who of course did not come right away and by the time he got there and dosed her she was ready to push. It was so hard for me to sit there and watch my friend suddenly lose control, in so much pain, and not be able to help her. She kept saying, "I can't do this, I don't want to, it's too much pain". I wanted to get in her face and tell her she could do it, that she had to get control. I wanted so bad to tell her what helped me through the contractions, but I soon realized that even if I told her exactly what I did to get through the contractions, it wouldn't work. She wasn't prepared to deal with it because it just hit her like a freight train out of nowhere. Anyway, Luckily, one of the nurses told her she had to listen and get control if ONLY for the baby's sake. So she was able to focus a little better and push for the baby's sake. The baby had some trouble breathing for the first day and my friend was very frustrated because while she FELT the entire delivery starting from when she was dilated to an 8, including the tear and stitching, her legs and lower body went completely numb afterwards. Go figure. I watched as they offered her painkiller after painkiller once it was over. I thought about how amazing I felt after (our daughter) was born, how strong and happy and relieved I felt. Yah, I was still in a little pain, but it didn't phase me.

Well after I left the hospital, I went home, my mind racing, thinking about the question her husband asked, comparing my experience etc. Today, I started researching birth statistics, and natural birthing. I did a lot of research like this before I ever got pregnant. That research led me to YOU. Anyway, I am just amazed. I am amazed by all this information and I once again, found confirming to me that natural child births (for healthy individuals) are more successful when it comes to not only mortality of babies and mothers, but overall birthing experiences and outcomes. I am amazed that the risks for using technology for birthing are SO REAL yet ignored, while all this information about natural birth success is completely ignored. I am amazed that this information I have just found today in 30 minutes is not made known to people. I am amazed that more women don't do their own research. I am amazed that I sometimes feel SO nervous to talk about my decision for natural child birth to people because I am afraid people will think I am crazy or stupid, while deep down I KNOW it was the right decision. I am amazed at how many people told me I was crazy for doing it while I was pregnant and told me that I would never forgive myself if something bad happened. I am sorry I didn't respond by saying "I would never forgive myself if something bad happened as a result of a technological resource at the hospital, because the stats show more bad things happen to women who give birth in hospitals than to those who don't". I am so frustrated that I wasn't prepared to properly defend myself or communicate to people the confidence I had in natural childbirth during the many times when my friends and family questioned me. The only person who I felt completely supported me (besides my husband) was my mother in law, and for a good reason, she birthed her babies in the hospital, but refused epidural's. During the birth of her first baby, the doctor was pressuring her to have an epidural, but he didn't know that her placenta always detached too early and for some reason (I don't really understand) the epidural would have caused serious problems had she gotten it. Anyway, that doctor later came to her and told her she would have lost the baby had he given her the epidural.

Sorry for the ranting, I guess I just need to put this in my journal. The only thing I really need to say to you, Donna, is that I appreciate you SO much. I am so thankful that you have followed your passion and beliefs in natural health to become who you are. I am so grateful I was able to find you because you are rare.

Love, Melissa

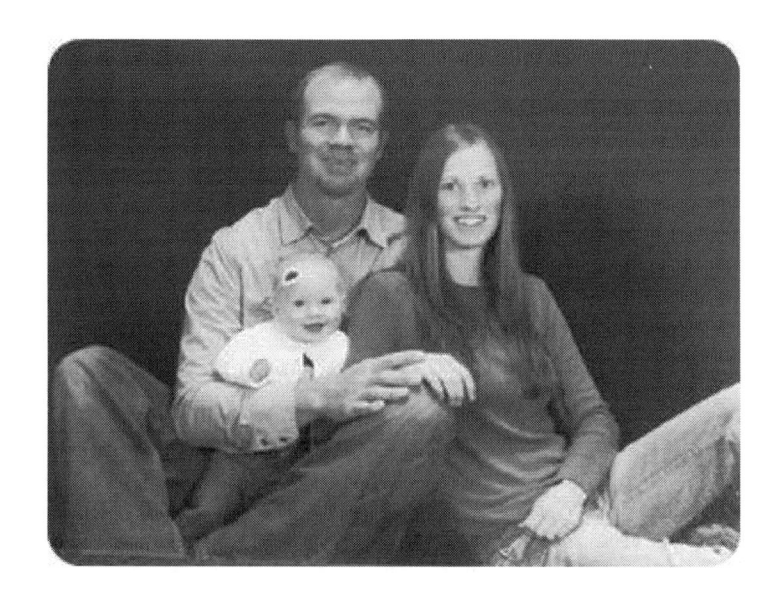

~20~
LABOR AND DELIVERY

The labor and delivery process is a mystery to most people, men and women alike. This section is to teach you what is going on, what steps the body takes throughout and what to expect from a home birth situation. Keeping in mind that all birth attendants have their own style and technique (mostly depending on what type of attendant it is) but if you are prepared with solutions of your own then the process can go more smoothly. Remember, that this is not support for UCB (Unassisted Child Birth) because of the increased chances of complications caused by inexperience and this is not intended to be a guide to UCB. This section is a continuation of your personal education.

Start of Labor
When labor starts it will, generally, form some type of a pattern. The contractions will usually start out with a twinge that lasts about 10 seconds and comes back every 20 minutes or so, then the twinges will get to where they last longer and come more frequently. By the time they become "pains" they are usually lasting 30-40 seconds and are down to 5-6 minutes apart. By "transition" the contractions will be at their height of intensity and generally have 90 seconds in between each contraction and last for about 90 seconds. This is the average labor pattern. Depending on diet and lifestyle, this can take from a couple of hours or less, to a much more extended time. False labor will not have a pattern and will not progress.

Cervix
Contractions during labor are caused from the muscles of the uterus pulling the cervix open. The cervix is the gateway between the uterus (a flexible bag-like organ that holds the baby during pregnancy) and the birth canal (vagina). If the cervix is not open then the baby cannot descend down into the birth canal to be born. The length of time that it takes for this process varies but the healthier the woman is, with proper diet and exercise, the shorter the labor time will usually be. The longest labors I see are in the girls who insist on eating breads throughout the pregnancy or have 'spectators' in the room.

If a woman is lying down on her back, the cervix, prior to pregnancy is straight back to the end of the vagina and feels somewhat like the end of the nose. The cervix sticks out about as far as the end of the nose and is of a similar texture. It will have a small hole in the center (round if she has never given birth and curved like a tiny smile if a woman has had a baby slide down through it). The muscle of the vagina feels more spongy as the woman nears time to deliver. The vagina relaxes in order to prevent the muscle from tearing as the baby descends down the birth canal.

Effacement
Effacement is the thinning of the cervix. Dilation is the opening up of the cervix. The cervix, prior to labor, will become less thick and then will begin to open up. Women vary, but most will be dilated to three or four centimeters and more than 50% effaced prior to the onset of contractions. If the cervix is thin when she begins labor then the cervix will respond to the contractions by opening up more easily due to the lack of resistance of a thicker cervix and this results in a shorter labor time. The opposite circumstances will also hold true, if labor is induced prior to proper preparedness, one can expect to have a long hard labor with an increased chance of a c-section or other complications.

Patterns
In the early part of labor you may prefer to get up and walk around or rather be busy doing something. During this time you will most generally need little or no attention. You will probably

feel in control and enjoy the process of knowing things are beginning. Staying hydrated with wholesome fluids is important. Equally important is the frequent check of yours and your baby's vitals. The fetal heart tone and your pulse and blood pressure should be taken to insure safety of both. If you get dehydrated or your blood sugar, or blood pressure drops, you can fatigue and the chances of an emergency increase. If your blood pressure drops then electrolytes or licorice root are most commonly used. If the blood sugar drops then I have my girls eat wholesome foods or take licorice root. This is generally not allowed in a hospital.

When things get more intense, if allowed, you will fall into your own pattern. Some women may want to walk during the contractions, others will want to lay or sit, but the one thing that is common with most is that the contractions will reach a point that they will require her entire concentration to work through them. This is a time when she will hear what is said, but will be unable to respond until the contraction ends. The majority of the time between contractions should be spent resting instead of chatting or answering someone else's unnecessary questions. This is your time and you are the one doing the work so you should be the one making the choices. You may want people close, or you may want people out of the way. You may be talkative or quiet, but whatever you choose, if not risking safety issues, your desires should be allowed so that labor will go smoother for you and your baby.

Spectators
I have found that if there is one, or more, person in the vicinity that a mother is not comfortable with, is antagonistic or otherwise threatening to our laboring woman, she will not progress. Even having people she loves and generally feels comfortable with can delay labor. This tends to be a primary reason for failure to progress with dilation and effacement. Privacy needs to be upheld. The more people there are the more often we see complications. Someone who I have grown very fond of said it well when she said "It was a private matter that got you into this mess, and it takes a private matter to get out of it". As a birth attendant, I watch our expectant mom, and her interaction with other people around her, during the weeks prior to the birth. If there is someone that brings on snide remarks or causes the mother to shut down positive emotion, then I watch this more closely. If I have a 'failure to progress' then I ask the husband to remove all 'spectators', no matter who they are. If they fail to leave, or stay gone at his request, then I remove them for the birth area.

I had a group of women at a birth, who all had good intentions, but they were loud and laughing while our lady was laboring and she stopped progressing. Another had about 20 people out in the yard and next door waiting for her to birth as well as 2-3 in the house and she stopped progressing. Another had two very nice, and mostly quiet women waiting in the other room and she stopped progressing. All of these ladies failed to progress, past four or five centimeters, in their current environment. All of them dilated quickly after their environment was cleared (except for husband and birth attendants) and had their baby in their arms within 90 minutes.

Comfort
Once you reach a point of having to concentrate you should never be left alone, as things may take a while or they may happen very quickly. Through contractions you may need more support. At this point there are several things that can be done. Every woman is different and different techniques should be encouraged until the right one is found.

Your support person can clean out the bathtub and run it full of very warm water (Adjust the temperature that is best for you). The bathtub should be filled with enough water to cover as much of your belly as possible. If your water has broken, then adding a ¼ cup of rubbing alcohol can insure there are no bacteria in the water. You can situate yourself into a position that is the most comfortable for you whether it is on your back, on your side, sitting up, and etcetera. As you lay in the tub, your mate, birth attendant, or support person can pour water over your belly and breasts. Some women like this between contractions, others like it during contractions and others like it during both. Listen to your body and politely direct for what is best for you. The warm water will help to relax the muscles to relieve pain. Most women enjoy labor for a while in the bathtub and as long as it feels good to you then keep it up just be sure to have someone with you while you are in the tub.

Sometimes, due to hormones and extra work, a woman will feel over-heated during labor. This is a good time to use a cool washcloth to wipe your face with in between contractions. Until the baby is born, a fan or open window is acceptable. Once the baby is born then these need to be stopped as you do not want to chill your baby.

Pressure Points
The divots at the bottom of your back, just above the tailbone and off to each side of the spine, are good points to have pressure applied to during labor. Some ladies like to have their husband stand in front of them with his arms wrapped his around her. Usually, the natural place for his hands to rest is right over these pressure points. If he can slide his fingertips into these spots and apply steady, firm pressure (without rubbing or massaging them) during a contraction it may help with the pain. If you are more comfortable squatting, kneeling, sitting or on your side then your support person can use the thumb and index finger of one hand to apply pressure on these divots during the contractions. Guide them to the exact spot, as well as the amount of pressure, that feels best to you.

The feet also have pressure points to assist with comfort during labor. Exactly mid-way between the ankle and the point of the heel, on the inside of the foot the pressure point for the uterus can be found. The pressure points for the ovaries can be found on the outside of the foot in the same place. At the top and center point on the sole of the heel is the pressure point for the cervix. If you put your foot up so that your support person can take the heels of your feet in their hands, they can put the thumb on the inside point, the tip of the middle finger on the outside point and the knuckle of the index finger on the pressure point for the cervix. You should know immediately if this is something that is going to work for you. If the points are found and pressed correctly, a positive change should be seen in the first contraction. Your support person should let go of them in between contractions or if it does not make you feel better.

On the inside of the leg, approximately an average sized woman's hand width directly above each ankle, there is another point used for cervical dilation. During contractions this point can be pressed to help speed dilation and assist in pain relief. Use if it feels better to do so.

If you feel pressure in your legs with the contractions then squeezing the muscles on top of the leg, above the knee during contractions will also help in alleviating the pain. This can be done by the support person or by a laboring woman, if she has the strength. The first couple of contractions will tell if this is right for you.

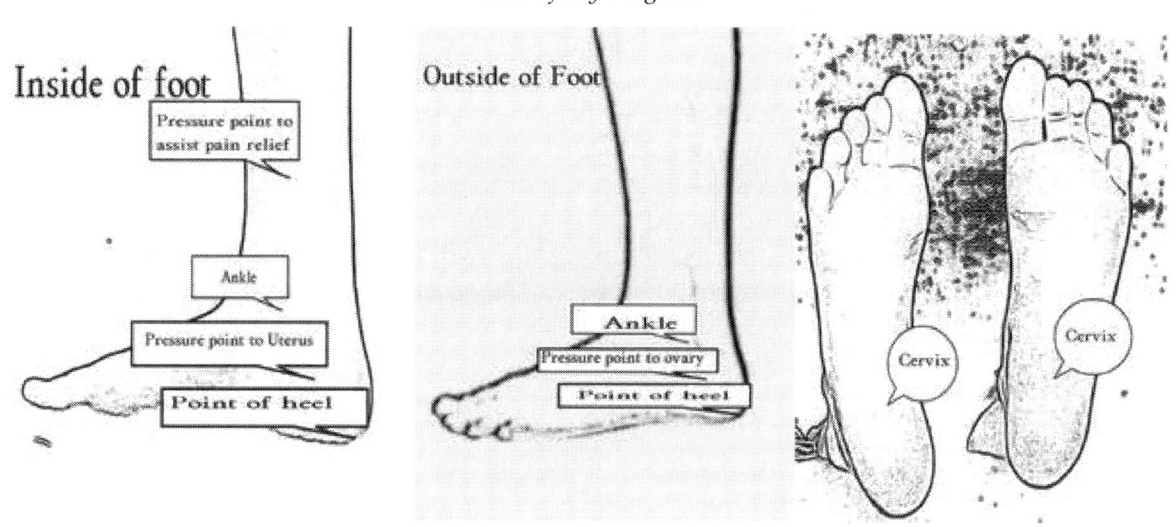

After the contractions become more intense, if there is more time, then hot packs can be placed on the back and lower belly. This is done by heating water to about 180-190 Fahrenheit and having your support person, with gloved hands, dip clean tri folded wash clothes into the hot water and lay one across the divots in the back and another just above the pubic bone in the front. If it is too hot in the beginning, just cool it a bit by flipping it in the air for a few seconds then try again. Change the clothes between contractions, not during. Just before transition, most women really like using hot packs, but once you are fully dilated and ready to push then continuing the packs is usually not possible.

Pushing
Once the cervix is fully dilated it will move back and disappear completely into the bottom of the uterus, increasing the size of the muscle at the top of the uterus to assist in the pushing process. If there is a ridge (also called a lip) on the cervix, you are not fully dilated and need a while longer to complete the process which usually only takes a few minutes.

If a woman pushes before she is fully dilated it can cause the cervix to swell, may result in the failure to progress any farther, or can even tear the cervix resulting in 1) a bleed at the birth and 2) a scar to form on the cervix, so that it makes dilation hard and sometimes even impossible during any following pregnancies. It is essential to wait until you are dilated completely or the baby can be felt in the birth canal before pushing.

Once the cervix is fully dilated the baby's head (assuming baby is in the proper, head down, position) will slide into the cervix. As the baby's head penetrates the cervix, there will usually be a small show of blood, this is just a few drops, similar to a small period, called 'active show'. Shortly after the blood show, within another couple of contractions, the mother will generally state that she has pressure that feels like she needs to have a bowel movement. This is caused from the baby applying pressure to the lower bowel as baby moves down the birth canal to be born. If there are any signs of excess bleeding we start immediately on shepherd's purse tea, one teaspoon in a cup of hot water cool if necessary. Drink with a straw if possible. A dose of, Ferrum Phos. 6X cell salt #4 is also given every 10 minutes if necessary (found in most natural health stores).

If there is low back pain, from a low back or tailbone injury, then you can either move to a birthing stool, go into a squat or just roll over onto your side. If you have had a low back or tailbone injury, lying on your back to deliver is usually not as effective because the tailbone is unable to float out of the way increasing discomfort and slowing the progress of the delivery.

As baby descends down the birth canal there may be a small amount of stool show up from the mother. The stool is actually a sign that baby is making progress because the stool will appear at the same pace the baby is moving down the birth canal. If the stool is showing very quickly, it tells you that the baby is moving quickly down the birth canal and the perineum needs immediate support. I generally have 4X4 gauze pads, toilet paper or paper towels to move the stool out of the way and drop it into the garbage that is within arm's reach. If the stool appears a little at a time then one knows the baby is moving slow but making steady progress and this may be a reason to move into a better position. By changing to a birthing stool, squatting or kneeling position then gravity is working with her body and the baby will descend more quickly. If the decision is made to change positions, do so in between contractions.

As the baby slides down into the birth canal, if there is an additional birth assistant there to provide gentle rectal support then it will assist in preventing hemorrhoids. A little extra support prevents problems later on. Rectal support is just enough pressure being applied with a piece of toilet paper or paper towel to prevent a hemorrhoid. No more than a few ounces of pressure are needed. This assistant's hand needs to be kept out of the way of baby's head, during rectal support.

Crowning
While baby is crowning (baby's head can be seen from the perineum) checking the color of the baby's head tells how baby is holding up. If the baby's head is pink, baby is getting plenty of oxygen and is comfortable. If baby is turning red then baby is feeling a little pressure, but is still doing fine. If the head is a purple color then baby is stressed and things need to progress faster and this is when a mom should be placed into a squat or onto a birthing stool in order to assist the baby's descent. If the baby's head has turned blue then baby is unconscious and will need to be resuscitated after he is born. If his head is white then there is a floppy, lifeless baby and baby is going to need immediate attention or is stillborn. Depending on circumstances, the changing of colors can happen quickly so this is something to watch closely. It is always preferred to have a baby born while still pink and strong. Red is the next most acceptable. If any of the other stages begin to appear, then the process needs to be quickened by changing the birth position of the mother, in order to protect the baby. By taking mom off her back or side and putting her into a sitting or squatting position, gravity helps to assist with the process and she is not reliant solely on her strength to push baby out.

Once baby has crowned, and his color looks good, the baby's head and mother's perineum should have constant support by your birth attendant. An attendant will usually apply gentle counter-pressure back on baby's head, with the palm of the hand, as a woman pushes baby down the birth canal. As long as a woman is making low groans or cries, the baby is progressing at a pace that is comfortable for the mother and it is not at risk of tearing the mother. If the tone changes to a high-pitched cry (this is usually for a short time) or states, "It is burning" then baby is in the process of causing damage to the mother. The birth attendant will probably apply more counter pressure to the baby and calmly instruct mother, "Stop pushing, now". Waiting until the next contraction. During this short break, the body will rapidly send muscle relaxants to the area and it will be prepared to make more progress by the next contraction.

Dilation of the Perineum
As the baby's head progresses then a woman's body will stretch out over the top of the baby's head and the ears and nose can be felt and the birth attendant should continue with gentle support until the mother's perineum slides completely out of the way. The baby's head is dilating the perineum just like it dilated the cervix. This dilation of the perineum may take a few more contractions, but is worth getting baby birthed without damage to the mother. If it takes more than a few

contractions to accomplish this, the mother should have additional oxygen by either supplementing her oxygen and / or cooling the room and letting her wipe her face between contractions, with a cool washcloth, if she desires. If the mother is getting more oxygen then so is her baby. Drinking good, cold water between contractions also helps. (Chlorinated water has less oxygen than un-chlorinated water.) Note: If baby is losing color then it is worth risking a tear on the mother to preserve the life of the baby. Mother can be sutured later, either by the attendant or through transport but needs to be done within the first 12-24 hours, the sooner the better after mother and child are both stabilized.

The Cord
Once baby's head is completely birthed, the attendant should have the mother stop and relax while the cord is being checked (a woman should have from 60 to 90 seconds between contractions at this point to prepare). A birth attendant will more than likely gently slide one finger down around baby's throat to check for the cord. If there is no cord around the throat then the mother will be allowed to gently push baby out with the next contraction or sooner if she desires. As the birth attendant supports baby and encourages the mother to use a strong, controlled push to gently lay baby into the birth attendant's hands.

If the cord is around the neck then the attendant will try to move the cord up over the baby's head. If it is loose then it will move easily. If the cord is tight around baby's throat, the attendant will most likely slide two fingers of one hand between the throat and the cord to protect baby's throat and vocal cords from the umbilical cord. Then the mother can gently push baby on out. This may cause the placenta to be pulled away from the uterine wall while baby is being born and treatment for a bleed should be expected immediately after the birth.

Baby's First Breath
As soon as a baby is delivered the birth attendant will insure baby takes his first breath. Baby can be held upside down with the arms allowed to drop over the head to allow for the lungs to move, triggering first breath. I prefer to let baby lay on the bed or towel, on the right side, while taking a clean, dry towel and taking a quick and gentle swipe across the face to clear away fluids from the nose and mouth then gently, but briskly rub the little chest and back simultaneously. The brisk rubbing of the chest and back massages his lungs and heart to stimulate his first breath. Once baby is breathing comfortably, I lay baby across the mother's tummy with baby's head a little lower than the body to let gravity help move any extra fluid.

If the assistance of a bulb syringe is needed, then I lay baby on his right side and suction the lower side of the throat. Gravity will pull the fluid to the bottom side allowing the upper part to accommodate air passage. A birth attendant will usually clear out the throat and the nose with the bulb syringe by squeezing the air out, and by inserting it into the area expected to have fluid and then release to have the syringe extract the fluid and then will repeat this processes until all airways are clear. Any signs of purple or bluing show that a baby is not getting adequate oxygen and any blow by oxygen given should not be directly placed into a baby's face or nose, if there is not an infant regulator. Too much oxygen at a time can cause permanent damage to a newborn. Gentle 'blow-by' is preferred by putting the oxygen on a lower setting and slowly moving the tube back and forth from out past the face on one side to under the nose and then on past to the other side of baby's face. This actually puts over half of the oxygen out into the air around baby with less going directly into baby's sinus. The gradual increase in the oxygen helps support baby with better circulation.

In most cases, baby will be placed on a mother's tummy facing the mother (if the length of cord allows for it), with baby's head slightly down hill so that any fluids in the baby's mouth or nose can drain out of the body instead of down into the bronchial / lungs where it could potentially cause pneumonia. Baby is laid facing mother so they can see each other and get that precious eye-to-eye contact. Making sure the cord is over the top of baby's hip not pinched underneath baby allowing for continued circulation.

I generally leave the cord attached until it has quit pulsating. I am aware that this is a controversial issue and both sides feel equally strong about it. The reason I allow the cord to stop pulsating before it is cut is; the cord provides a back-up source of circulation and oxygen, to baby from the mother, until baby is stabilized. Waiting for the cord to be cut is a natural way for a baby to get the added support needed until the lungs are functioning properly. Once a baby no longer needs the support from mom then her body will stop sending circulation to the baby and will begin to release the placenta. This is the way nature intended.

After the cord has quit pulsating, I clamp the cord in two places, to prevent mother or baby from hemorrhaging. I use sterile hemostats to clamp the cord, however it can be just as effective to tightly tie it off with clean shoelaces or a strong, clean string. Anything going this close to a newborn needs to be very clean, and sterile if possible. Then the cord is cut between the two clamps. Once the cord is cut, then we wrap baby into a clean, dry towel. To be kept warm until the placenta is delivered and baby has a chance to latch on to nurse and bond with Mom.

Note, if there is an emergency with mother or child, I will cut the cord and get them separated so the one in need can be worked on without restrictions. Emergency situations call for emergency measures.

Delivery of the Placenta
No birth attendant should ever pull the placenta out of the mother in a home birth situation. Again, this is a controversial subject. The placenta is one of the most amazing things on this planet. It screens and separates foods and attempts to select the best of the foods for baby and then sends that nutrition to baby through two vessels that feed baby, directly, without going through the stomach and digestive tract. The placenta regulates the amount of naturally occurring antibiotics needed by baby and sends immune builders also. It does a wonderful job of screening out most infections and disease. It takes the wastes from baby and sends them back out to the elimination of the mother to be sent out of the body. It also regulates nutrients for proper cell division and growth regulating hormones that are needed for baby. It does all this and more from a 'stand still' position in the uterus where it takes up minimal room, leaving more room for baby and never putting toxins out to mother or child.

The placenta is an oval mass that generally weighs an average of one and a half pounds. One side of the placenta is attached to the uterine wall with a network of blood vessels going to and from mother while the other side of the placenta has the baby, attached by the cord, and is incased inside of the amniotic sac. During the birth of the baby, the amniotic sac usually breaks and baby descends down the birth canal and is then outside the mother while still attached to the cord. Inside the uterus, the placenta continues to pump blood to the baby until baby's lungs are stable and then it ceases to pump.

Once the cord is drained of blood then the mother's body gets a signal that the placenta is no longer needed. When the baby begins to nurse, the nursing action starts the uterus to contract again, releasing the placenta. The placenta slides down to cover the cervix and stays there, damming the outlet until any bleeding, that is coming from the site where placenta was attached, is stopped. Once the bleeding stops, then the uterus will contract to push the placenta out. In this manner the placenta is passed without risk to mother or child. This entire process usually takes 45 minutes to an hour, but can happen earlier. The medical profession is far more fluent than I in business and to them time is money. They are also organized to make the best use of both time and money. Even though most doctors will admit that it causes less scaring and less bleeding to let the placenta deliver naturally, they will also state they can stop a hemorrhage in less time than it takes to wait for the placenta. They are also in a position to stop an induced hemorrhage. They are trained and have the necessary backup to handle things more efficiently. A person may not have a choice to wait for the placenta in a hospital to detach on its own unless prior arrangements have been made with a birth plan in place. If you are at home, you are not in a position to have the placenta pulled out prematurely.

After the baby has been delivered and the cord quits pulsating and is cut, there should be a minimal amount of blood loss. The uterus will still be swollen and the placenta can be felt through the mother's abdomen as a hard lump. By rubbing a mother's uterus gently, but firmly the uterus will contract back down to its pre-pregnancy size in a couple of days. If her baby is latched on and nursing, this will also help stimulate the uterus to contract. When a mother gets the urge to push the placenta out she should do so with a soft, gentle push to avoid causing any damage inside the uterus where the placenta was attached. There is usually a small gush of blood after the placenta delivers, but it should not be more than about a cup. If a woman is lying down, it can take over an hour for the placenta to be delivered. If a woman's blood pressure is good, she can have help getting to a toilet, or a birth stool, to sit for a few minutes and gravity helps the placenta move down. If a woman ever gets weak, she should be helped back to the bed immediately. Black cohosh is an herb that has a strong estrogen effect, which causes the uterus to contract and giving her a couple of droppers of a black cohosh extract can assist in bringing on the needed contractions. Soymilk, 16 ounces, has been known to have the same effect as black cohosh, if the mother feels up to drinking that much. The placenta will be set aside to be checked by the birth attendant later.

Clean-up
The mother should be cleaned up with a washcloth and some warm water. Great care should be taken in cleaning a woman right after birth because she will be tender. A feminine pad, a pair of underwear and a clean top will usually be placed on her and then she should have the chance to eat and rest, but should never be left alone.

Checking the Placenta
The placenta should have an oval shape with veins that run through the side that has the cord attached. The placenta needs to be examined to make sure all the veins on that side of the placenta are there and that there are not any missing pieces. It should be a dark red color and should not have green, black or other colors. The placenta should not have a foul smell of infection and should smell of clean blood. The texture should be firm and easy to hold with one hand. If the placenta drips or tries to fall apart then it lacked proper nutrition and mom needs better nutrition during the next pregnancy.

The amniotic sac is attached and generally folded over the side with the cord. The sac is about the same thickness as a water balloon. The cord also needs to be checked. There should be three vessels going down through the cord. If there are only two, then it implies a possible heart problem. If baby has problems holding color and there is a two-vessel cord then baby should be seen by a health professional insure everything is okay.

Reasons to Transport
If you have access to phone service then your birth attendant should call ahead to let the hospital know you are transporting and a brief description of the problem so that they will be prepared for you upon arrival, limiting wait time. Always remain calm. The hospital does not want to hear accusations or hysterics they want an honest presentation of facts. At this point you have already determined that the problem is out of your control. Once you are at the hospital then you need to conduct yourself in a positive manner and trust them. They are now the ones in control.

Premature Babies and Underweight Babies: Premature babies are those that are born more than four weeks prior their due dates (no matter size). Underweight babies are babies born under five pounds and both should be transported as they could have under developed lungs or other organs. Babies born more than four weeks before their actual due date are not developed enough to be cared for by anyone without experience. Babies that weigh less than five pounds have special needs and are best cared for in a medical facility, if possible. If a baby weighs less than five pounds when born, he may lack the strength to latch on and nurse.

Prolapsed Cord A cord in the birth canal ahead of the baby is reason for a transport and should not be handled in a home birth situation. Once the cord is in the birth canal and the baby's head penetrates the cervix, all oxygen is shut off to the baby, giving a very short time to get baby out without losing him. Most babies take more than two minutes to pass through the birth canal (push time). Do not risk it. Placing a mom in a knees and chest position and transporting immediately will allow for baby to slide away from the cervix allowing baby oxygen until mother can be transported. (*Here is a diagram of knees and chest position*)

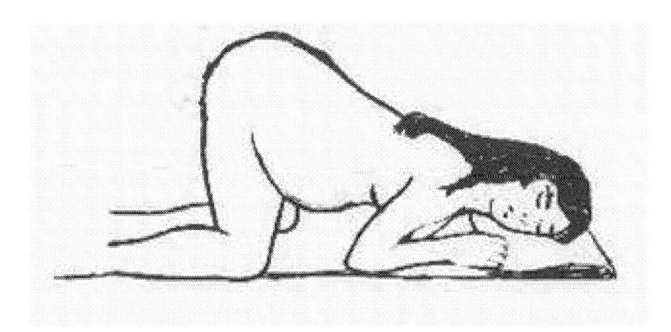

Excessive Bleeding Is another reason for immediate transport. If there is going to be a transport then a mother should be placed in a position where her heart is below or level with her uterus. She will bleed more heavily while sitting up than she would while lying down. Have her talk to her body and remain calm. Put ice on the outside of the uterus and either call 911, or transport immediately.

Placenta Previa Bleeding, prior to the birth, could be a sign of the placenta being low enough in the uterus to be blocking the cervix. If the placenta is covering the cervix there is no way for the baby to be born without medical assistance. A partial placenta previa can be delivered by an experienced birth attendant, but if there is any doubt about the percentage of the placenta that is covering the cervix, transport.

Breech Births Should not happen if a woman has followed directions listed under the third trimester section. However, breech babies should be in the hands of an experienced birth attendant as there is an increased chance of complications and they do need to be handled properly to avoid the danger of losing baby. Transport if at all possible.

High Blood Pressure If the blood pressure is over 160 on the top or 100 on the bottom then a transport is probably in order. Especially, if the blood pressure is rising or there are any symptoms such as headache, irritability, pounding in the chest or dizziness. BP should be taken often and transport if there is any doubt.

Irregular Fetal Heart Tones If baby's heartbeat is irregular, and not responding by giving oxygen to the mother, then it shows baby is probably under stress and is going to need extra help at birth. Fetal heart tones should always be strong and regular.

Problems where you are not in Control then you should either get someone there with enough knowledge to handle the problem or transport. The life of a mother or child should never be compromised.

A Word of Advice

Anytime you transport, you need to remember that you transported because there was one or more issues that you were not in control of. Once you transport you need to trust in the person and place you were transported to. Cooperate with them and try to work with them for a positive outcome. Remember that you were not in control and that is why you transported, do not attempt to tell them how to do their job.

Patient's Rights

If something happens that makes you feel this doctor is prejudice or inept, you are entitled to a second opinion. All hospitals have a Patient's Rights handout that lets you know what your rights are. (Keep in mind that your rights in a community hospital are going to be different than those in a private hospital so get a copy of the rights for the hospital you plan to go to in advance or upon arrival.) If you feel your rights are being violated then talk to someone immediately, but do not go into a hospital thinking you have the right to tell them how to do their job, that would be reckless. The Patient Rights list is a balanced set of rules that are to your advantage as well as for the hospital's protection. It is good for all concerned. *(Next is an example of a Patient's Right's form)*

You have the right *to participate in the development and the implementation of your health care plan.*
You have the right *to make decisions regarding your care.*
You have the right *to have a family member (or representative of your choice) and your own physician notified promptly of your admission to the hospital.*
You have the right *to request or refuse treatment. You do not, however, have the right to demand treatment or services deemed medically unnecessary or inappropriate.*
You have the right *to have your personal privacy respected. You have the right to request that visitors be asked to leave prior to an examination and when treatment issues are   discussed. Privacy curtains will be used in semi-private rooms.*
You have the right *to create an Advance Directive, which will help us comply with your wishes when you are unable to speak for yourself.*
Your Advance Directive or Durable Power of Attorney for Health Care *will be placed in your medical record so that your physicians and nurses will know what you would like done and who will make decisions about life support and medical care if you cannot make them for yourself. If you do not have an Advance Directive or a Durable Power of Attorney for Health Care and would like one, ask the Registration Department for the necessary forms.*
You have the right *to receive care in a safe setting, free from verbal abuse and harassment.*
You have the right *to confidentiality of your clinical records and the right to access information*
(Continues on next page)

contained in your clinical records within a reasonable time frame (except in certain circumstances specified by law). You have the right to be free from restraints and seclusion of any form used as a means of coercion, discipline, convenience, or retaliation by staff.

You have the right *to be treated with respect and dignity and to receive comfort when needed.*

You have the right *to file a grievance and to file a complaint. You may do so by: Requesting to speak with the Charge Nurse and/or Manager of the nursing unit, or writing or calling our Patient Relations office.*

~21~
BREAST ISSUES

I am going to begin this section by simply telling you that, "All breast milk is not created equal!"

When a woman's milk comes in, generally about 48 hours after the birth, it is not uncommon to have an over-production until the baby and mother's bodies adjust. The amount of estrogen in the mother plays a role in this also. Usually, but not always, there will be more milk if the baby is female because they are both producing the hormone, estrogen. The breasts can be so full that it causes pain because the baby is not able to consume as much as the mother is producing.

To Relieve pressure
Put about a tablespoon of castor oil on a washcloth and put it over the skin of breast and nipple then cover with a warm heating pad. This is usually very effective in reliving the pressure that is causing grief. The average time the heating pad is left on is about 30 minutes, but we have had ladies who slept through the night with the oil and heating pad on. Just listen to your own body.

Understanding the system
If milk is backed up into the lymph nodes then the gland under the arm (in the armpit) will be swollen. This tells us that the over flow passage ways that run into the stomach are blocked. To resolve this problem we need to understand the passage way because the body has to eliminate this naturally. There are passageways that carry the cerebrospinal fluid down the sides of the back of the neck, across midway to the shoulder and then down to above the center of each breast. Above each breast there is a junction (pressure point) where the extra fluids from the pericardium and lungs meet with the cerebral spinal fluid. (A) Then goes over and down to the outside of the breast under the arm, where it meets with the second passage causing pressure point (B) in diagram I... The second passage that takes fluid out of the arm, down beside the breast tissue (where it joins the first passage at (B) and straight down to the bottom of the rib cage, then up along the bottom rib to the solar plexus and to the stomach. At the curve of the rib directly below the breast there is a third pressure point (C) that carries the fluids, respectively, from/ around the liver or spleen and into the stomach.

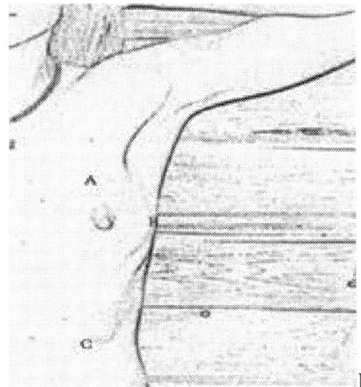

Diagram I

If any of the pressure points are blocked then everything before that is stopped up and probably swollen, causing pressure and pain. If the pressure point is blocked then it will be tender when touched. Stagnant milk held at 98 degrees is going to become infected from the natural bacteria that can cause a breast infection if left without attention. Thicker milk is higher in butter fat and is more prone to cause a blockage in the beginning.

If there is redness, either in patches or in lines, or if there is heat then one can expect that there is infection. Pain with baby latching on, is another indication there could be infection in the breast. Green or red colorations of the milk show possibility of infection or blood. When in doubt, I would treat for infection.

To Resolve the Problem
The following massage is best done by the ones spouse, if accessible. If he is not available then an immediate family member, like mother or sister, is the next best to do this work. It is a little difficult for a woman who is in pain to do it herself but it can be done.

To assist the body in moving off the excess milk, the passageway needs to be opened up and the milk redirected. Using olive oil as a lubricant, very gently use two fingers and rub the three pressure points in a small circular motion (about the size of a nickel). At first these will be very sore so be gentle. Spend about 15 seconds on each pressure point moving from (A) to (B) and then to (C). Again, gently start at the upper heart on the left and gently rub along the passage line from the upper heart to point (A), then down to point (B) and down the ribcage to the bottom of the rib moving up and over point (C) to the solar plexus and down into the stomach...as shown in diagram II. Then go back to the top and start at the point midway between the neck and the point of the shoulder and gently rub down to point (A) and then over to point (B) and keep following the same pathway on down into the stomach. Repeat each of these steps two to three times. This will assist in opening the passageways.

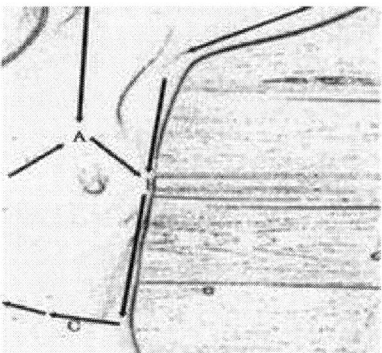

Diagram II

Once the passageway is open, the breast is still going to be very tender so be careful. The breast has two hemispheres, the upper and the lower. It is important to always work in the direction of the natural flow of the body and not mix the hemispheres or move backwards. Start on the inside of the upper hemisphere next to the breastbone. Again with olive oil to lubricate, very gently rub from the inside of the breast out towards pressure point (B) as shown in diagram III. Do not touch the nipple or the areola. Then take it down along the same passageway as when opening things up and take it to the stomach. In the beginning you will not touch any heavier than if to rub only the skin level, do not try to go deeper into the breast. Repeat the same process with the lower hemisphere by starting at the breastbone and working out towards point (B) and then down and to the stomach. Repeat alternating between hemispheres. This is done four to five times before moving to the other breast and following the same technique on that side working a mirrored pathway as you have done on the first. As the massage is repeated the breast usually becomes softer and there is less pressure allowing the massage to go a little deeper but never should it be massaged deeper than about ¼ inch, not trying to disturb the glands underneath.

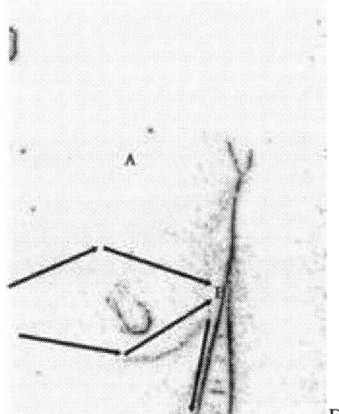

Diagram III

By taking two droppers of 500 to 1100 ppm colloidal silver, orally, with each massage treatment usually helps rid the body of any infection that is there also. The massage treatment is repeated every 45 minutes or so for about five to six hours. If the colloidal silver is not available or is not working for the given situation then seek attention for the issue. If left unattended most infections will continue to grow.

Adjusting Butterfat Content of Breast Milk
Even though thick (yellow) milk has more substance and is very satisfying to baby, mom may have a few more issues with it. Thin milk leaves baby unsatisfied and will usually need to nurse more often, never really being content. The key is to balance the thickness so it is comfortable for mother and child.

If the milk is too thin, it will have a white or blue tint to it. Eating a handful of raw almonds or cashews will increase the amount of butterfat within an hour or so. Make sure there is plenty of healthy fats and proteins in the diet. The fats should come in the form of raw nuts, avocados or olive oil. Proteins can be best obtained by choosing meats and beans, but never by drinking protein drinks that have amino acid isolates in them. Amino acid isolates are not meant for mother/infant consumption whether directly or through breast milk. Most amino acids / proteins should be derived from whole foods.

If the milk is too thick, it will have a heavier consistency and will have a yellow color to it. If this is the case then the mother needs to drink more clean water in order to dilute it. Try to drink either spring water or purified water but avoid distilled water as it has had all the minerals removed. Increasing the water content will result in less fat per ounce than undiluted milk.

Some moms will eat a handful of raw nuts in the early evening to help increase the butterfat to give baby more substance to make baby feel more satisfied. This increases a baby's chance of sleeping through the night. A small dose of high quality calcium (not from a rock base like coral, egg shell, oyster shell, bone meal etc.) at the same time can also help baby to relax, after baby is 6-8 weeks old. "I Love helping those little ones rest through the night, it makes life better for baby and parents!" Avoid any foods that cause gas as these foods can cause colic in baby. Sugar in a mom's diet can cause thrush and diaper rash in baby as well as add to the possibility of a yeast infection in mother's breast.

Loss of milk supply
For the mom who is not able to sustain her milk production at any point, raw mammary gland in either glandular or low potency homeopathic (such as 6X) has run a beautiful success rate. Taking it on an, "as needed" basis. Be sure to drink plenty of water and eat plenty of meats, vegetables, and

fruits.

Supplements for Breast Issues While Nursing

- 500 to 1100 ppm colloidal silver for bacterial infections.

- Goldenseal root for bacterial infection (not for anyone with low blood sugar).

- Caprylic Acid, not soft gels, for yeast infections.

- Broad based friendly flora (acidophilus with at least 8 strains) after any type of infection to replace friendly bacteria in mother and child.

- Mammary gland, raw or homeopathic (low potency), to increase milk supply.

- Soymilk to assist with estrogen for increasing milk production.

- Black Cohosh to increase estrogen for milk production (Too much black cohosh will result in a headache in the center of the forehead. Cut back or quit if a headache develops).

- Sarsaparilla to decrease milk production.

- Blessed Thistle to increase circulation into the breast, Marshmallow root to mildly increase milk supply.

- Sage and parsley are used to decrease milk supply.

Never go hungry while breastfeeding. If you are not eating then your body can't produce milk. Eating healthy proteins, fats, fruits, grains, vegetables, and water help to produce healthy breast milk that is critical for babies. While breastfeeding, your intake of water needs to be increased.

Never take diuretics while nursing. Diuretics will run the fluids back through the kidneys, bypassing the breasts and cause a loss of milk production.

If a food causes you to get gassy then it will usually cause baby to get gassy, resulting in colic. Sometimes foods will upset baby that will not upset your system. Foods like chocolate, cabbage, radishes, sugar, spicy or acidic foods are all known for causing colic. Each child has his/her own system, but if your baby has an upset stomach then you need to closely examine your diet to locate the problem. After all, if he is exclusively breastfed then all of his nutrition is coming from the foods that you are ingesting. If you keep a journal of the foods you eat and the times your baby gets a tummy ache, it will not take long to figure out the culprit. It took me less than a week to figure out that the problem in my diet, for one of my babies, was mustard. Yes, there was nothing in common with the main course or side dishes and the only common denominator was mustard. Once I stopped eating foods that had mustard as an ingredient, he never had colic again.

Eat enough fresh fruits. If you are eating enough fresh fruits to keep your bowels open then your baby will have fewer problems with his bowels.

Diaper rash in breastfed babies is usually caused by the mother eating sugar, yeast, milk or wheat. Removing sugar, yeast, milk and wheat from your diet and giving baby some kind of friendly bacteria should cure the diaper rash. When it comes to the different brands of pro-biotic (friendly bacteria) the only thing that I look for is one that has several different strains and can be dissolved in fluid. A ¼ teaspoon dose of pro-biotic mixed in a liquid twice a day should allow you to see improvements within a few days.

I called one of our ladies a while back to make sure everything was all right. She told me that she was doing fine but the baby had suffered colic for a couple of weeks and she would start crying after the evening meal and would not stop until one or two in the morning. Baby also had a terrible diaper rash for about the same amount of time. So I asked, "Are you not following diet?" "No," she replied. "After my six week checkup I started eating breads and sugars again." "Okay, that is probably where her problem is. Go back onto diet and start taking high potency friendly bacteria and see what happens." I told her. She agreed and I called back a week later to see how things were going and she told me that baby had no diaper rash and stopped being fussy about three days after going back onto diet. She told me, "I feel terrible that I was eating the things that were hurting her. I won't go off diet again until she is weaned, I don't want her to pay that price." Wise move!

If you are stressed or upset when you sit down to breastfeed then baby is going to be very prone to getting a tummy ache from the milk. Drinking a cup of chamomile tea, taking some calcium or just taking a deep breath and relaxing will help. Breastfeeding should be a time for mom and baby to bond and is a nice way to take a break away from the other issues of the day.

A couple of years ago I sent a couple of questions out to a few of our ladies regarding breast milk and this is what they had to say...

Ladies,
The questions I would like to get feedback on are...
1) If there was (hypothetically) another mother, within our group, who was unable to breastfeed for any reason would you be willing to donate your extra milk to help that baby?
2) If, (hypothetically) there were a problem that took your breast milk, would you be willing to use milk from another mother, within our group who was following diet, for your baby? I would like to hear all sides of this issue... Please give me feedback.
Donna

Hey Donna!
The answer to the first question is yes, as long as I had extra to give, I would be more than happy to do so. I feel breast milk is the best for babies. The answer to the second question is also yes, of course, providing the other mother has a good and healthy diet. Human milk is always best for human babies!
Blessings,
JM

If there were a need, I would fit in the extra time to pump extra milk. Staying hydrated and using herbs to encourage milk production if needed, I'm sure that double-duty would be do-able for any period of time during the next two years (I'd up my calcium and iron etc.) And if something happened to me and I couldn't feed my two month old, I would be so grateful if someone would do that for my baby until he was, say, 6 months old and could transition to goats milk and pureed veggies, etc. If mother's milk were not an option (we would be willing to pay a lot for it if it were), my husband would research like crazy until he found the absolute best formula out there and pay and arm and a leg for it. Nutrition is a big deal to us, and while their bodies are still developing so fast, it's interesting that the majority of Americans appear to do well on a formula-fed start, but as long as we

could give them better tools, we try our best.
WR

Hey Donna,
If I am able to breast feed I would be happy to supply my breast milk to another mother in our group. For the second question, Yes I would love to have someone give us their breast milk if they are following diet and are healthy if I'm not able to breast feed. I want the best for my baby!
LR

I know how hard it is to have to put a baby on a bottle instead of nursing. I dried when my first two babies were only four months old. At that point and time I would have loved to have mother's milk to give them and I would have never questioned the mother's diet.

I have learned a lot since then. Donna suggested some herbs when I had my third baby and I am happy to say I finally enjoy nursing for the first time. My milk never dried up with my third, forth or fifth. It really surprised me because I started thinking that I was just a woman that would have to accept that nursing wasn't possible for me. However if there ever came a time that I could not nurse my baby I would love if another mother would be willing to share (that is if she is following diet). As for me I would be willing to share in a heartbeat.
EO

I would greatly appreciate if someone who had the same diet and feelings as myself were willing to feed my child if my milk dried up. I would also offer that same service to another mother, since I have more than enough.
RD

Hmmm, Well, the western snooty side of me would say, eeeewwww! However, the much more primal motherly side would say if the situation calls for it, I'd want what's best for my babies and other babies, too. I think I'd sooner donate to someone than have to hire out a wet nurse for one of my kids, and I guess I'm thinking this would be a fairly serious situation, not an any day "got milk?" type thing. I'd never want to think of anyone's little one starving...Our culture doesn't suit to such ideas, but if the need be... I guess we'd have to change our thinking on many fronts. I have always liked your idea of an herbal alternative of some sort of broth and tea mix, but not if the real deal were available....
EB

One morning I received a phone call from a woman who told me she was adopting a baby and she wanted to breastfeed her new baby. This would have sounded questionable under most situations but this lady threw a new challenge into the picture. She was in her 50's and had been going through menopause for about 5 years and the last time she had given birth was 18 years earlier.

I would have thought this an impossibility except that my father, who was very gifted with livestock and natural health had taken a mare that had not had a foal on her in several years and got her to produce milk for a foal who had lost it's mother. I thought "Well, if Dad could do this with a horse, we should a least give it a try for this new mother-to-be." I asked her when the baby was due and how long we had to prepare her body. With the excitement of a new parent she said, "He was born about 6 hours ago!". "Oh my goodness! This is short notice," I thought. She was very religious and very devoted to her intent to breastfeed. I looked up Father's recipe and changed it a bit to fit this woman.

Here was Father's recipe.

2 pts. Marshmallow
2 pts. Comfrey
2 pts. Slippery Elm
1 pt. Blue Cohosh
1 pt. Blessed Thistle
1 pt. Red Raspberry
1 pt. Dandelion

This is what our lady took (in addition to her faith and regular prayers for His help) several times per day.

2 caps. (1/2 tsp.) Black Cohosh
2 caps (1/2 tsp.) Red Raspberry Leaves
2 caps (1/2 tsp) Marshmallow root
2 caps (1/2 tsp) Blessed Thistle

And she took this 3-4 times per day along with lots of water and red raspberry tea. Within a couple of days she was starting to lactate, within 10 days she was breast-feeding and shortly after she needed minimal supplementation. She continued to produce mother's milk for her son until he was 3 months old. How wonderful!

Notes_____

_____

_____

_____

_____

_____

_____

_____

_____

_____

_____

_____

_____

~22~
ELIZABETH'S STORY

I had 4 pregnancies in hospitals with allopathic medicine. Three different hospitals with three different doctors for the 4 pregnancies. I don't have a weight problem until I get pregnant and then with each of those pregnancies I gained 50, 55, 60 lbs and it would come off eventually, most of it. I would just get so big and with that comes a lot of discomforts. Eventually your joints start aching and you don't have any energy. They put you on prescription prenatal vitamins but I didn't feel any improvement with those. I was just fatigued a lot of the time, I think just having all the extra weight. There was no explanation as to why, just goes without saying that while you are pregnant you are going to put on this weight. It was just expected. So there was no reason why and there was nothing you could do about it. It was just "Yeah, that stinks, huh?".

You have problems like ligament and joint pains and it is to be expected. They'll say "Well, you need to start expecting this now" and they'll tell you why. You understand because you are growing and there is no help for it. Then they send you on your way. I feel like its kinda treated like everybody knows what to expect. Everybody's heard the old wives tales "Oh, yeah, I got so big when I was pregnant" and "Oh, I ate this bad and I had these pains" and there's no question it's just expected, that's how it is meant to be. When you are pregnant you are going to feel tired, you're going to be fat and you're going to have no energy. You need to be in a doctors care and you need to deliver in a hospital.

I remember reading with my first pregnancy and it was a radical book written around the time I was born in the 70s, when they had all the women's liberation propaganda. They talked about childbirth and I remember something, they said " Pregnancy is not a disease but we treat it like its an illness" . It stuck with me. I thought "This is what our body is meant to do so why is it so difficult? Why am I having all these aches and pains? Why am I so exhausted?" I remember trying to do simple things like trying to get in and out of a car, I felt like I needed a forklift. It was just a really difficult situation trying to do anything. I was just tired all the time. I think that was the big thing, the endless naps and sleeping.

Infections, I never had yeast infections in my life until I was pregnant. Again, there was no explanation as to why they were happening. They would just say "Yeah, this happens, this is to be expected. This is OK, this is common. This is normal". When is disease normal?

The first time, the only time, I had a bladder infection, I honestly didn't know what was wrong. I went into pre-term labor and had to be hospitalized. My doctor was out of town and the doctor on call was pretty upset with me because I was only twenty-some-odd weeks along and ready to have the baby too early. The baby was barely viable at that point. The doctor said "Aren't you having frequent urination?" I said "Sure, but I thought that was normal." The doctor said "Don't you have any back pain?" I said "Yeah but they told me that was normal." So I didn't know I had an infection. I didn't realize that anything was wrong. Needless to say, they were pretty upset with me. I had to spend a couple days away from my family at a great expense. I never had these things when I wasn't pregnant so it put me in a mindset that "When you're pregnant your body is weak. When you're pregnant your body is tired. When you're pregnant your body is more prone to disease. That is all normal and that's all good and fine".

I remember when I first started seeing Donna. She came at me with "OK, here's the situation. This is the way I do things. These are the things you can eat. These are the things you cannot eat." I thought "That's bizarre" because never before had anyone talked about diet and what you should and shouldn't be eating. She was very, very concerned about sugar. I thought "OK, well, everyone knows sugar is not supposed to be a health food. Alright." Then there was the issue about bread and I thought "Well that sounds a little harder for me". I've never had a big sweet-tooth. The sugars didn't panic me and I didn't think the breads would be a problem. So I said "Sure, OK" and I thought it was a little off but surely what you eat doesn't matter. I know back in the day people used to say "You are what you eat" but nobody says that anymore. You eat what you doggone well want to and the doctor is supposed to have a pill for that.--to fix whatever the problem is. It just never occurred to me that what I ate mattered. Really, I knew you were supposed to get your vegetables and your fruits when you're pregnant and I did. I didn't have a problem with weight. I've never been a 'junk food queen' type gal. So I said "No problem" and I went home.

I remember looking around my kitchen and pantry. I had just gone shopping and all the cupboards were full. I remember crying to my husband and he said "What's the matter?" I said "There's nothing to eat." He said "The kitchen is full!" I said "I know, but I can't eat any of it and I don't know what to do." It was very hard, I hadn't realized how big a part, flour products-in particular, were in my diet. In everybody's diet. Sugar for that matter, was in things I never dreamed had sugar. I didn't believe it at first. It was mind-blowing to me that if I didn't eat these things I was not going to gain a million pounds the way I usually do. I'm not going to get the infections that I always had and I had always lived with. It was a revolutionary idea and I just couldn't believe the words coming out of this woman's mouth. "If you don't want to be sick anymore, if you don't want to gain two million pounds, if you don't want the infections, don't eat the garbage." I thought "Where does she get this stuff? Nobody talks this way... they usually say "Eat for two!". It was a real mind-blowing thought that it could make that big of difference.

When I tried it, I thought I could do it. I thought it was going to be easy. I had never had big food addictions--I didn't think-- until I tried to get off of flour products. That was very hard for me. I didn't realize how often I ate pastas and breads. I was actually really into it and I ended up calling her a few days later. She said "How are you doing?" I said "I am a bread addict, that's all I eat!" I didn't even know. She told me it was critical. I tried it and the more off of those things --the more I didn't eat those foods, refined sugars and breads--the better I felt. I didn't gain 50-60 lbs anymore. My energy level, the vitamins she put me on, I felt like a human being again. I had more energy on her program with my fifth baby than I had not being pregnant, period. I just couldn't believe it was possible, I thought "If I feel this good while pregnant with my fifth child, imagine how I'd feel not pregnant at all! Just following her plan, the nutrition intake". There is a big, big difference in the supplements she gave and the prenatal vitamins your doctor would give you. Huge difference, night and day.

I have always read a lot. I remember asking the doctor with my second pregnancy "What about additional supplements? What about these other kind of supplements?" He said "You know what you're gonna have, Honey? You're gonna have expensive pee. Really pretty, bright colored, expensive urine. Don't waste your money." So I never did.

Donna put me on all this stuff and I thought "Well, here it is" but I felt good, I had energy! That is really important when you are pregnant with number five because you have four other ones to keep up with. I just felt good, I didn't have the problems I had before. I didn't have infections anymore and I didn't feel sick all the time. When I followed diet, my joints didn't ache. I didn't get heartburn so I wished I was dead. I could lay flat in bed, on my pillow, at night and not feel like acid was being poured down my throat. The ligament pains, she had something for that. The nausea, morning sickness, she knew what to do about that. She does not expect that you are to be sick and miserable and uncomfortable, overweight and diseased while you are pregnant.

I remember when I delivered my babies and began nursing, my body kind of knew 'OK, we're through with the baby part' and I'd get so sick. Later on in the week I'd break out with a fever, with an influenza. I never had uterine infections just the crud--flu, cold, respiratory, junk. I remember Donna calling to check on me after one of my births and she said "How are you feeling?" I said " I'm sick, you know, I just have this going on. No, it's not uterine. I'm fine, it's my sixth baby and I'm over 30 now." She said "Elizabeth, have I taught you nothing? You don't have to be sick. This is not normal. It's not normal for you to become terribly ill because you had a baby. Having a baby is perfectly normal, perfectly natural. You should feel good. You should have no disease at this point. This is not a justification." She told me what to do. Which is the beautiful thing about it. She has answers. That's the thing I love most is 'There are answers!'.

I delivered my 8th child two weeks ago today. I gained 20 pounds, all of which were shed by my ninth post-partum day. My total labor was about 3 ½ hours long and without any complications. This has been typical for me on this program and I have more energy, less illness and each of the children are peaceful and vigorous. I am so sold on this program that I not only use it with each pregnancy but I have put my entire family on the dietary guidelines, herein recommended. My husband who had suffered many heath conditions, before we met Donna, has since lost 40 pounds and is no longer on any prescription medications that we believed he would be on the rest of his life. All eight children suffer far fewer illnesses than any others I know. As for me, I am healthier as I approach 40 than I was in my 20's and I will continue to use this program long after my child bearing years are over. We are grateful for Donna's knowledge and are happy to make 'healthy' our new lifestyle.

~23~
ERIN'S STORY

My last pregnancy was riddled with problems and I felt ill constantly. I had at least three migraines that landed me in the hospital for IV fluids to combat dehydration.

I went past my due date so the doctor decided to schedule me for induction--on my birthday. I wasn't nuts about the idea of being induced, but arrived at the prescribed time, was placed on the monitor only to find out I was having regular contractions. The doctor decided to go ahead and start Pitocin to accelerate the process, what ensued was significantly worse than with my first child eight years prior. I ended up having an emergency c-section after laboring all day. My baby was not tolerating labor well, and the doctor told me it was because he was face presenting and had a short cord. I was exhausted and in immense pain for the next several days, my husband was traumatized from the whole experience, and my baby looked like he was in a boxing match. Shortly after my pregnancy I was diagnosed with Hashimoto's disease. I struggled to achieve normal blood levels of thyroid hormones, and reduction of symptoms, for over a year. Just after I turned 28, I found out that I was expecting my third baby. Feeling a little shell shocked from my last experience I wanted to take a more natural approach. I had read the testimonials on Donna's site after stumbling across it one day and was ready to do whatever it took to have a healthy pregnancy and happy baby. After my first call with Donna I decided that I wanted her to be my pregnancy advisor, while the local doctors took care of the "prenatal care." I have not regretted a day since! I never felt bad about my food and lifestyle choices, but once I started following Donna's advice my life changed dramatically. I stopped writing off my symptoms to pregnancy and started feeling better than I had in years! I am amazed at how the OB doctors seem so surprised that I am doing so well and they have actually encouraged me to keep it up because it is obviously working. I have yet to end up in the hospital with a migraine (and have actually had significantly less headaches) and I have lost about 10 pounds to date, and gained a healthy growing baby that I cannot wait to meet! I feel AMAZING and could not have done it without your wisdom and encouragement Donna.

*** Baby Dylan was born and 6 days later, Erin sent this letter******

Despite having an enormous list of things to accomplish today I thought it more important to sit down for a few and send you an update....and a huge THANK YOU!

Dylan had his first well check yesterday and is doing fantastic! We see the doctor whom I used to nurse for. While in the office I was astounded at the number of compliments I was getting from my former co-workers, not only for having a super cute sweet baby, but at how well I was looking and feeling. I remember new moms like myself coming in for that first check looking as tired as can be, in sweats and visually in some degree of pain--NOT ME! We went in early to pick up a friend and go have lunch before our appointment, and I was looking and feeling suitable to be in public.

I have way more milk than this poor little guy can handle, feeding ad lib and still able to pump 12+ ounces at least 3 times a day. We are so fortunate for this as I am able to not only share feeding duties with the rest of the family, but I should have a nice cache frozen for my return to work where I may not always be near to go over to the infant care center and feed and snuggle with him.

I am SO glad that our paths crossed and that even from afar you were able to play such a key role in my pregnancy. I do not by any means believe that the standalone care I would have received from the OBGYN's would have ended so blissfully. Surely I would have been bullied into a c-section (and still recovering from that), even the first doctor to come in and see me was skirting around the "c" word, I had the courage to stand up to him and say he needed to come up with a plan B as there was going to be no c-section happening on this girl today...Thank God for the on-call rotation, I ended up with the one doctor that I have been seeing more so than the others because he stood whole heartedly behind my decision and did everything in his power to give me this (I'm going with divine intervention on this one). While Dylan's arrival was not everything I hoped to provide for him, I believe under the given circumstances that I was able to do a pretty darn good job because of our relationship, and the knowledge you armed me with. It may not have been the perfect L&D but definitely stood out above the previous two. I actually have to admit that I am somewhat disappointed that it was my last, but pleased that it ended on a high note.

Lots of love,
Erin

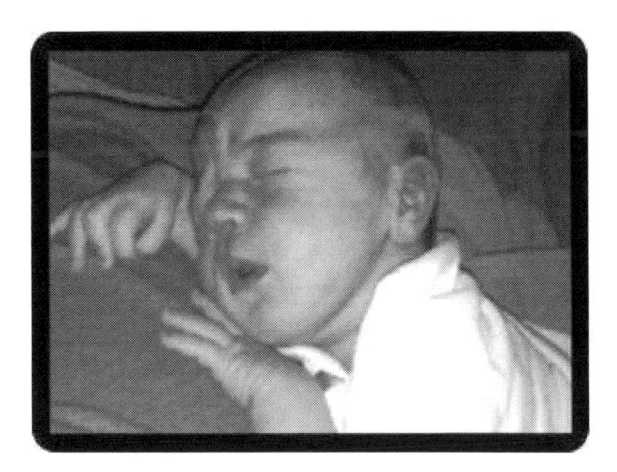

~24~
BABY AFTER THE BIRTH

This section contains things that most health care providers check during the first few minutes after birth up to a few days after birth, and a few tips and tricks that parents can use to help their baby. *Note: Understanding that all babies are not boys, I refer to baby as 'him' and the mother as 'her' for ease of reading and to avoid confusion.*

APGAR
When babies are born we expect them to show signs of health and vitality, the APGAR is a nice quick overall assessment of the newborn baby. The first check is done at one minute, the second at five minutes, and the third is at 10 minutes after the birth of the baby.

The APGAR test was devised by Dr. Virginia Apgar in 1952, and is used in all hospitals and birth centers and is required by the State to fill out birth certificates and this is how it works.

Appearance, Pulse, Grimace, Activity, and Respiration are the areas noted and each area is given a score of 0, 1 or 2. A perfectly healthy and strong baby is going to have an APGAR of 10. Score is noted as follows.

APPEARANCE
0 if baby is blue or pale all over.
1 point if baby is pink with bluish extremities (hands or feet) 2 points if baby is pink all over
2 normal color all over, hands and feet are pink.

PULSE
0 if baby has no pulse
1 for pulse under 100
2 for pulse over 100

GRIMACE
0 for no response to stimulation
1 for grimace or feeble cry
2 for strong healthy cry

ACTIVITY
0 for no muscle tone
1 for some flexion
2 for flexed arms and legs that resist extension

RESPIRATION
0 for no breathing
1 for weak, irregular gasping
2 for strong, healthy cry

If the APGAR test ever shows lower than 6 then baby should be in the hands of a professional for emergency care. If born at home and the condition of baby is deteriorating, by these standards, then a transport is strongly recommended. (This holds true with older children, also.)

Documentation
The date, exact time, sex, APGAR, gestation of baby when born will all be turned in for the birth certificate and is always nice to keep in a journal. After baby has had a chance to nurse, bond with parents, and things are quiet then the birth attendant gives the newborn a final exam by checking the following.

Weight should be checked with accuracy, preferably right to the ounce or gram. It is essential to have the baby's accurate weight so if any complications arise they can be detected early. If baby starts to dehydrate, it will be in ounces lost, not by amounts large enough to determine by sight or by pounds. I like to see babies between six and seven point five pounds at full term. If dietary instructions are followed, the weight will generally fall into this spectrum and babies are strong and healthy without the added stress on mother or baby during the birth process. Babies that weigh under, five pounds five ounces, need to be seen by a professional.

Length
Length is determined by measuring from the top of the head to the bottom of the outstretched leg. Most at term, or near term, babies are between 19 and 21 inches long at birth.

Head
The size of baby's head will vary depending on the mothers diet during pregnancy. When dietary guidelines are followed, the size of an average baby is about 14 inches. When dietary guidelines are not followed, a baby's head can reach up to 16 inches, or even larger if there has been large amounts of sugar, flour, and carbonation consumed during pregnancy. The measurement of the baby's head should be within a half inch of the measurement of the chest.

Chest
The baby's chest is measured at about nipple level and should measure within about ½ inch of the head measurement. Having the chest measure significantly smaller may be of some concern. A smaller measurement is usually from lack of nutrition while developing in utero or could show a potential risk for hydrocephalus (fluid on the brain) and while the latter has several causes the primary cause is viral. If the chest is significantly larger than the head then it could show a growth malfunction and should be checked to insure everything is fine with baby.

Vernix
While baby is in utero, his little body is covered by a white, waxy, cheese-like coating, called vernix. Vernix is considered to be a protective coating for the skin, containing anti-bacterial properties and is generally seen more on babies that are born a couple weeks before their due date. When a baby is full term, he tends to have less vernix, and it can usually be found on the lower back, under the arms, behind the knees, and under the neck. When a baby is past full term (a little over due) there is usually no vernix left and the skin tends to be dry. Applying olive oil to the skin is usually very healing and can make baby more comfortable.

Skin
Baby is looked over for any signs of missing skin, rashes or other signs of abnormalities like lumps, lesions, moles, pustules, birth marks or bruising. It is not uncommon for Hispanic, African American, Indian, or Asian babies to have a blue marking that looks almost like bruising called Mongolian Spots. Caucasian babies can have them, but it is not common. Mongolian Spots are not associated with disease or illness and are considered normal for those races. A gentle touch can test to see if baby is sensitive, as he would be with a bruise, and if the spots are not sensitive they are probably not a concern. While these problems are rare, any concerns or questions should be

taken up with your health care provider.

The Head (skull)
A baby's skull is made of bone plates with soft spots in between. The soft spots between the plates are called fontanels. The fontanel on the top of the head is the largest and shaped like a diamond. The second fontanel is on the back of the head and is smaller and triangular in shape. These fontanels are thin, flexible pieces of membrane and are what make it possible for baby's head to slide down into the birth canal during birth. These soft spots will eventually disappear (be filled in with bone) around 9-18 months of age.

If the plates of the skull seemed to be fused tight and there are no 'soft spots', this is usually due to the formation of the cranial sutures or in the more rare event of abnormal brain development (abnormal development rarely occurs if a woman has adequate nutrition during pregnancy). A small or absent fontanel can lead to headaches later on in childhood and after baby is a little older you may want to have him seen by someone who does cranial work (a type of massage) for plate adjustment. It is a very gentle process and babies are usually content to be worked on.

If the plates that make up the skull are more than three centimeters from touching then it can show either a lack of Vitamin D, low thyroid, or hydrocephaly (excess fluid around the brain) and should be checked by a care provider.

If the baby spent only a short amount of time in the birth canal then his head is usually pretty round in shape.

If time in the birth canal was prolonged with a long pushing time then the baby's head can be misshaped and most of this will usually subside in a few hours. Occasionally, there can be a small pocket of fluid that forms between the skull and the skin that feels soft and may be sensitive to baby. This fluid will generally reabsorb into the system over the next 60 days or so, but any tenderness will be gone in a few days. I generally use a lavender and olive oil mix to rub on the head to help disperse the fluid and help relieve any sensitivity. (Ten drops lavender oil to one ounce of olive oil dilution--then use like lotion) Run fingers along the base of the skull and along the jaw line very gently to look for protrusions or any other abnormalities. If there is a sign of a mass or a lump in the fontanel or along the skull or jaw line then it is always a good idea to have baby seen by a professional.

Eyes
A newborn's eyes should be alert and focused within a few minutes of birth, if the light is not too bright in the room. A newborn's eyes are usually sensitive because of the lack of light in utero and after newborns have had anti-bacterial drops put into the eyes they will not be able to focus as well. Giving baby a chance to have direct eye contact with parents not only assists with the bonding, but it also allows your health care provider to watch the baby's ability to focus and control eye movement. Your health care provider will most likely; gently tip your newborn up and down to see if his eyes will spontaneously open and close. Watch for the newborn to track with his eyes as people move or as baby is moved. Observe for signs of being cross-eyed and make sure that both eyes are working together without a jerking motion.

Baby's First Cry
When a baby cries, the cry should be clear and it should be a strong cry. Usually any fluid in the throat or nose can be removed with a bulb syringe. By laying baby on his side and suctioning the inferior (lower) nostril leaving the superior (upper) nostril for breathing. The same is repeated to clear the throat. When a newborn's cry sounds weak or is short, with a 'grunt' at the end it shows

a problem that needs to be seen immediately by a medical doctor as this can be a sign of respiratory weakness.

The Sucking Reflex
By sliding a (preferably gloved) clean small finger (the pinkie) into the newborn's mouth with the nail down and the pad up, your health care provider can feel the roof of the mouth to ensure the palate is complete. It should feel like the roof of your own mouth and should not have holes, lumps, or abnormalities. While checking the roof of the mouth, baby will generally suck on the finger, giving a chance to feel the strength of the sucking reflex, which should feel strong enough to extract the colostrum from his mother. While the birth attendant is there, there will be a check for any sign of a lip deformation. The palate and lip have a direct impact on the baby being able to latch on and nurse.

Breathing
Baby should breathe comfortably through the nose with the mouth closed and without any sign of congestion (fluid) in the nose. This can be checked when baby is nursing and if baby is breathing through the mouth or has to break away from sucking to catch breath then extra time should be spent trying to remove any fluid from the nose. If there was a meconium show in the amniotic fluid (making the water green) then your care provider may use a 'delee' to suction the baby to lessen the chances of pneumonia.

The breathing of a newborn should be very quiet and shallow. By placing a stethoscope on the newborn's back and checking the upper, middle and lower section of the lungs at any place on either side of the spine, over the ribcage, a clear exchange of air should be audible. A rhythmic in, out, in, out, with just the sound of air should be heard without any crackling, gurgling, or any other sounds of fluid.

Other than looking for a clear air exchange your health care provider will also check for the number of times that baby breathes in one minute. 1 Inhalation and 1 exhalation are counted as 1 complete breath. The normal range is between 30 and 60 breathes per minute and is lower if the newborn is asleep. Grunts and difficulty breathing are signs of a problem and warrants concern.

Heart Rate
Baby's heart rate can also be checked using a stethoscope and should be within the range of 110 to 160 beats per minute if awake and slower (105-120) when sleeping. If the newborn's awake heartbeat is less than 100 beats per minute or over 170 beats per minute then baby, should be seen by a professional. The heartbeat should be regular without doubled or skipped beats. If it is irregular then there is an arrhythmia and baby needs to be watched. Sometimes hawthorn berry extract (glycerin) will regulate it but if it does not improve within days, seek a healthcare provider you trust for help.

Abdomen
Gentle fingertip massage of the abdomen is usually done to check for any potential masses or to find organs that do not fit under the ribcage. Any abnormalities show a concern and need to be checked by a professional.

Digestion
Intestinal sounds, that show there is activity in the intestinal tract and the baby's bowels are active, can be found by placing a stethoscope on baby's abdomen and listening for a gurgling sound. This gurgle means the bowels are working. Lack of gurgle is a concern.

The Back
Your health care provider will examine the back for any signs of abnormalities such as lumps, divots, breaks in the skin, or patches of hair along the spine. The most common cause for abnormalities on the back is what is called a sacral dimple, which is a small hole or divot off to the side of the spine, usually near the tailbone. This is a sign of a possible weakness that could have evolved into spina bifida. Spina Bifida is a defect of various degrees where the spine can grow on the outside of the body, as well as other symptoms such as hydrocephalus (fluid in and around the brain), paralysis, and/or limited mental function. I have found that children with a sacral dimple are usually a little harder to potty train as they tend to have a weakness in the elimination system that makes it difficult to hold their urine and sometimes stool. They also tend to run with a stiffness in the hips, which makes them a little less athletic than some other people, but generally does not restrict abilities. It does not seem to affect mental function or the personality and should be recognized and brought to a health provider's attention in any following pregnancies. If I have a woman who has ever had a baby with, or there is a family history of, a sacral dimple then I recommend taking a little extra folic acid prior to conception and during pregnancy. I also recommend taking an herbal supplement called skullcap that is to nutritionally support physical nerves. This, along with the rest of the prenatal supplement program, should give adequate nutrition to lessen then chances of a reoccurring or exaggerated problem.

Examining the Rectum
Examining the rectum helps to tell if it is complete. If the rectum has a layer of skin sealed across, so there is no opening, then baby needs immediate medical attention. If baby has had a bowel movement, the rectum is considered complete.

Meconium
Baby should pass meconium (first, black stool) in the first little bit after being born. Sometimes it is right after birth, other times it is several hours. If baby has not had a bowel movement within the first 18-24 hours the care provider will generally use a rectal thermometer, that has been lubricated with olive oil or water soluble gel, and insert it just past the sphincter muscle (about ½ inch). Then apply gentle pressure to the side of the rectal wall to bring on an urge to push the first stool out. When your care provider does this, they will be very gentle and not apply any more pressure than the weight of a nickel. They are simply trying to activate the urge for baby to push for a bowel movement and baby will push the stool out.

Checking Hips
Checking the hips is done by laying baby on his back and then gently taking his legs in hand and rolling the knees upwards toward his chest, while having the fingertips supporting the little hip joints, then gently rolling the knees outward to where they are moved into a butterfly position. Then gently bring the legs down together and straighten the legs out and repeat. The legs should move without resistance, discomfort nor clicking. Clicking is more frequent in female babies than male babies and can be a sign of an underlying neuromuscular disorder or a sign that the joints and muscles are not quite developed.

Checking Reflexes
Reflexes are usually checked by stretching out one leg and letting it rest in the provider's hand, when baby is relaxed, gently take a fingernail or end of pen and run it up the bottom of the foot, baby should pull his foot back. This shows his reflexes are developed. Check the other foot in the same manner. Generally everyone in the room will giggle when baby pulls his foot away. I have found this to be a perfect time, as a care provider, to hand baby to his mom, his daddy, grandma or whoever is moms support person (mother's choice) and let them dress baby for the first time.

Treating the cord
People in our society are accustomed to a cord taking 7-14 days to detach. The cord usually starts to smell bad and it can sometimes become infected. I have found that after the birth of a baby, if the cord is allowed to stay attached until it quits pulsating and the blood is moved out of the cord then it heals faster. Every time I have seen an attendant push the blood from the cord back into baby there has been an umbilical infection. Keep in mind that two of those vessels are taking blood and nutrition into the baby from the mother. The other one is taking baby's wastes back to the placenta to be sent through the mother's kidneys. When one squeezes the waste blood back into the baby they are sending it the wrong way. If there is any blood left in the cord, next to baby's body, then the blood should be squeezed toward the cord, not toward the baby, then clamped. Once the cord is clamped, cut and trimmed then the cord can be treated so it can heal in a reasonable amount of time. I take a 4X4 gauze pad and cut a slit about 1½ inches long in the center of it. Slide the gauze over the cord stump and then pour olive oil over the cord and surrounding gauze. Then fold the top and bottom edges of the gauze down over the stump. The gauze under the stump protects baby's tummy from the rough edges of the stump while the layers over the top protect the cord stump from the diaper and the olive oil helps to heal the cord. Once the cord is treated then baby can be dressed. The gauze should be changed with each diaper change and care should be taken, the cord will be sensitive and will start to hang loose before it falls off. DO NOT CUT OR PULL ON THE CORD, allow it to detach completely on its own. The cord will usually be healed by the time baby is about three to six days old. Any signs of redness, foul odor or gooey discharge are signs of infection. Watch closely. High potency colloidal silver dropped on the site can help to prevent infection, but I usually leave that to parental choice. Some also add essential oils, like lavender, to the olive oil treating the cord to relax baby.

Color
If baby has a nice color without any blueness or dark purple this is a good sign that baby is getting enough oxygen. Bluing shows that for one reason or another there is an inadequate supply of oxygen. When a newborn is blue your health care provider will first give baby additional oxygen, if it is accessible. If his lungs need a little extra help then this should do the job. The oxygen and gentle 'blow by' with the tube should never be held closer than 1½ - 2 inches from a baby's face and giving a newborn too much oxygen can cause irreversible damage such as blindness.

I also give about 100iu of d-alpha vitamin E. Vitamin E has been used for increasing blood oxygen for decades. However, remember that Vitamin E is an oil soluble vitamin, which means it does not break down in water, therefore a person can overdose from the kidneys not being able run off the excess. Vitamin E should be short term (not over a week) and no more than 100iu three times a day for an infant.

Lavender oil rubbed into the bottoms of the feet generally assists in helping baby's oxygen. Lavender works by increasing the circulation in the body.

If the heartbeat is irregular or color changes back to a blue color then hawthorn berries (in a glycerin extract form) for nutritional support into the heart. This is generally continued for the next six months to make sure there are no continued problems.

If none of these things bring his positive color in a short amount of time, or if the coloring worsens, then baby needs to be transported for emergency care.

If baby's color bleaches out or he looks pale (for the nationality) then this can be a sign of infection. It is generally bacterial, but is not worth the wait, don't hesitate to transport, especially if baby is not nursing well or is losing his body heat if unwrapped, such as in diaper changes. Infection can also show up in the color of stool and in the cord not healing properly. When in doubt have baby checked by your care provider.

Temperature
A newborn baby should be able to hold his body temperature, on his own, in a reasonably warm room for short periods of time, such as bathing or diaper changes. If he is getting blotchy or is turning colors then his temperature needs to be checked. This can be done by, wrapping baby up for at least 10 minutes and then taking his temperature. Then unwrap him for at least five minutes, in a comfortable room and then take his temperature again. If the temperature drops by even one degree then it is a sign baby is not holding body heat the way we expect. Keep baby bundled and watch for any other signs of concern. If there are any other signs of concern then contact your health care provider.

Holding Breath
The story about a baby or child holding their breath to get attention is a serious misconception, in my opinion. When a person inhales they are drawing in air through the pulmonary (lungs / respiratory) system and the oxygen is then converted into the cardiovascular (heart/blood) system. When a person exhales the body is letting go of the (left over gas) carbon dioxide through the pulmonary system. If a person inhales and then can't exhale (holding their breath) it is because that conversion of oxygen from pulmonary to cardiovascular is not being made properly. I have found that up to ¼ tsp of Hawthorn Berry extract on a glycerin base, three times per day works very well for most children. Ten drops three times per day for a newborn.

Breast Feeding
If a newborn is allowed to nurse (latch on) during the first hour after being born, the nursing instinct usually comes naturally and he tends to be more comfortable than if there is a longer delay. As soon as the cord is cut and sometimes before, if the cord is long enough, baby is placed skin to skin with his mother (draped with a clean, dry towel) and given chance to have his first feeding. The mother can be tired for the newborn's first feeding and having a pillow to support her elbow on the side baby is latched on, can be of great help so that she does not have to exert the extra energy needed to hold the baby up. While breast feeding, the baby is best positioned while lying with his belly facing mother's belly and with his mouth lying next to his mother's nipple. When baby opens his mouth to nurse, the nipple is slid into his mouth. The pressure of the nipple on the tongue will usually stimulate a sucking reflex and once he is rewarded with colostrum for nursing he will know what to do thereafter.

If the sucking reflex does not happen automatically, then gently rub the chin, while he is attached, directly below the center of his bottom lip and this will generally stimulate the reflex. Colostrum is the substance that comes in before the mother's milk and contains vital immune building, enzymes, anti-bacterial and anti-viral agents, and contains more oxygen than milk does. Once mother's milk comes in, it has fewer immune building agents, but has a higher fat content and is more satisfying. While there is very little colostrum produced it has high nutritional value. Babies usually eat less often during the first 48 hours after birth, making colostrum baby's best source of food and no supplementation is needed. Baby should be encouraged to nurse at least every four hours for a few minutes. After the first 48 hours his appetite will increase and he will want to eat more.

Umbilical Hernia
Umbilical hernia is usually caused from pressure being applied to the naval during the birth. This happens most often when the cord is wrapped around the neck or is otherwise tangled around baby. It can also occur if there is a shorter than normal cord that does not allow for baby to

descend without pulling on the placenta during birth.

In the days of old, they used bellybands, which were a belt of soft material (usually flannel) with a large coin set into the center to give baby's naval support. Sometimes it would give enough support to allow for the hernia to heal. If there are no signs of bleeding, infection, discoloration or other signs of immediate concern then many doctors will allow the infant time for the hernia to heal until the child is two or three years old. If there are any signs of infection, bleeding, discoloration or the hernia is getting larger then baby needs to be seen by a medical doctor. A belly band, with healing herbs, or poultices can give added support to ward off surgery until the child is older, but in most cases hernias are best taken care of medically.

Rashes and Irritated Skin
If a rash or some sort of skin irritation occurs in a breast-fed baby then a mother's diet should be closely looked at. When I see rash or eczema on a baby, I resolve it with a, long-term, change in a mother's diet because most skin irritations or rashes are caused by toxins. These toxins that should have been able to pass through the liver, kidneys, and spleen, take the next path of least resistance and come out through the skin. I always start by changing the mother's diet and then giving baby a pro-biotic to assist immune function which can help to heal any skin irritations or rashes. Using olive oil over the rash or irritated skin can also help to assist the skin's healing abilities without blocking the pores.

Diaper Rash even though it is, in most cases, caused from yeast which cannot be filtered through any of the organs, can also be solved by a long-term change in the mother's diet (no sugars, breads, or milk) and giving the baby a pro-biotic. If the baby's diet is being supplemented with formula than choosing a brand with less sugar or even a hypoallergenic formula should help. I would also choose a pro-biotic that contains bifid bacterium infantis and allow baby's bottom to air dry for a few minutes during each diaper change.

Cradle Cap
Cradle cap (seborrhea dermatitis) is not a sign of un-cleanliness, but is a sign of yeast in the body. If baby is being breast fed mom should stop eating sugars, breads, and milk to keep the yeast from thriving and some type of pro-biotic should be given to baby to help balance the friendly flora. The pro-biotic should contain several strains of bacteria, one of the primary bacteria should be bifid bacterium infantis, which is a friendly bacteria specifically found in infants.

Keep in mind that as long as you are in control and are seeing improvement in your baby's condition then you should stay the course with what you are doing. At any point that you do not have control or baby is not improving with whatever issue you are working with then contacting someone else is suggested. Depending on the situation you can either contact your healthcare provider or transport to the emergency room. If it is an emergency then immediate transport to the hospital would be advised. Older children and adults can speak to relay concerns but newborns do not have that ability so you must watch them closely for signs of concern and act appropriately.

Congratulations on your new little one!

~25~
MOTHER AFTER THE BIRTH

Things to Watch
After you give birth you need to be watched. If you are going to have a problem it is going to happen in the first 48 hours, as a rule. Watch closely for any signs of concern.

You should not lose your color from giving birth, no matter your nationality, you should maintain a natural and healthy color. When darker people start looking Caucasian, there is a problem. When Caucasians lose the pink from their cheeks, nose, and lips there is a problem. The problem in both cases is due from a loss of blood or a drop in blood pressure. A person with already low blood pressure can't afford the same blood loss as a person with normal blood pressure.

Avoid getting up if you are in a weakened condition as there may not be enough blood to reach the head area causing dizziness or unconsciousness. You should be resting until you have enough electrolytes and iron/vitamin K to stabilize yourself. Generally, blending 8 ounces of fresh spinach with fruit or juice and drinking it is plenty to stabilize a new mother after the birth of her baby.

For this reason, you should avoid walking with baby across the room for the first 24-48 hours after giving birth. You should spend your time, with baby, sitting or lying down. When you feel that you have your strength back, then it is safe to pick up baby and walk. You should have plenty of rest, even if you feel like you do not need it. Getting up (over exertion) too soon can increase the chances of a hemorrhage.

Having a loss of blood can also cause the milk to either come in early or not come in at all. Early change from colostrum to milk can result in baby not getting the proper nutrition, antibiotics, and oxygen from the colostrum. Lack of colostrum can affect babies immune and oxygen levels.

Your hormones are going to be different than they were while you were pregnant and so you will need to regulate the temperature in your environment. Sometimes you may feel colder and need more blankets and other times you may feel too warm and want less. Make sure that baby does not get chilled if you are over heated. If baby's skin feels even slightly cool to the touch then he needs to be bundled in a blanket.

New moms need to have plenty of healthy food available. Chicken broth based vegetable soups, preferably homemade, are usually full of nutrition. Meats, grains, and vegetables will give your body the proper nutrition to build strength while fruits will help keep your digestive system from being sluggish. Mothers, after giving birth need to make sure they are getting plenty to eat and drink.

During your first trip to the bathroom, you should have someone with you just in case you start feeling dizzy or weak. If you start to get lightheaded or weak, someone needs to help you get back to your bed immediately. It is not uncommon to pass a few clots upon standing or during your first couple of trips to the bathroom. There should not be an excessive amount of blood. Ferr Phos 6X can be given anytime there is an increase in bleeding. Sanitary napkins should be changed frequently, even if they are not full, to reduce bacterial buildup that could cause infection.

Urination is a good way to tell how the birth went. If there is a burning sensation upon urination then this is a sign of a tear or scratch. If there is a burning sensation following urination, a solution of; one ounce mild iodine solution to seven parts water mixed together in a peri bottle can be used to help rinse the perennial area. The mix should be sprayed on everything from the front all the way back to the rectum, including on the inside of the outer lips. This inhibits the growth of infection causing bacteria. (*This step would be skipped if a woman is allergic to iodine*)

Supplements after the Birth
I like to have my ladies take an herbal formula, starting immediately after the birth, that helps assist in preventing a uterine infection. I like to use one that has red raspberry leaves, blessed thistle, dong quai root, queen of the meadow leaves, marshmallow root and lobelia herb with a small amount of golden seal root. This formula has been very effective in strengthening a mother's female and immune systems to ward off any infection. The supplement I generally recommend is through Nature's Sunshine Products and is called FCSII. I recommend taking three capsules three times a day until the entire bottle is gone. If bleeding increases after quitting the supplement or there are any signs of infection then taking an additional bottle is suggested.

St. Johns Wort liquid (it needs to be a very dark extract) works with the hypothalamus to encourage the uterus to contract back down to its pre-pregnancy size as well as prevent postpartum depression. The support of St. John's Wort is most needed during the first 48 hours after giving birth. My recommendation for dosing is one dropper full each time baby is fed.

Note: St. Johns Wort is not to be used with any MAO inhibitor, as there can be major side effects. Do not change to St. Johns Wort from a MAO inhibitor but stay strictly with doctor's recommendation. St. John's Wort has also been known to cause sensitivity to heat. While on this product, avoid exposure to excess sunlight or heat. If exposure to sunlight or heat cannot be avoided then St. Johns Wort should be discontinued if sensitivity begins.

Continuation of the Super Supplemental is recommended but should be reduced to two tablets each morning. If the Super Supplemental is taken in the afternoon, the B-Complex in it could be giving energy to baby just as you are ready to go to bed and you do not want baby awake while you are trying to sleep. The Super Supplemental should be continued for at least six weeks after the birth of your baby. After that point, it is up to you to listen to your body and decide whether or not you still need it. If you feel better taking it, than not, then by all means take it.

A husband will usually benefit from taking two to four Super Supplemental vitamin's each day for the first couple of weeks after the birth. He is the one who catches the most physical damage after the birth because he is working, then comes home to take care of mother and child. Everyone seems to be watching over mom and baby, while father is in need of a little protection also. Extra nutrients during this time are a good preventative measure for him so he does not get worn down. This would hold true for any support person who is putting in extra hours to help with the new mother and child.

Prenatal tea should be continued for at least six weeks. It can be taken longer if there was excess bleeding or there was a tear at the birth. Some ladies drink the tea routinely for years to give nutritional support to their body. There is no reason not to but, again, listen to your own body.

Vitamin E should be continued for six weeks after the birth. This assists the body to heal without the build up of scar tissue. Colloidal Minerals can also be continued for at least six weeks after the birth of your baby.

Beyond supplements
Along with the herbal supplements the mother's uterus needs to be rubbed or massaged down to insure the contractions are working the uterus down to its pre-pregnancy size. If this is done

between each nursing then the uterus should be down to normal size the first 48 hours or so. The idea for rubbing the uterus is to stimulate the uterus to contract and without contracting it cannot shrink back down to size, which makes the uterus viable for infection and potential bleeding. Post birth contractions should stop as soon as the uterus reaches its pre-pregnancy size, which is about the size of your fist.

If you feel chilled, have a fever, have slimy or a foul smelling discharge, and/or heat or pain in the uterus, (not a contraction) these are all signs of a possible uterine infection. You need to be seen by your health care provider. Large doses of high potency colloidal silver and golden seal root (if you are not hypoglycemic) can reduce and even get rid of infection. Uterine infections are dangerous and need to be taken care of at the first sign of a problem, hence the reason we try to avoid them. If you don't start seeing results immediately then transporting is strongly recommended. Uterine infections usually do not happen until a few days after the birth, not in the first 24-48 hours.

If you had a hard delivery or did not have rectal support during the delivery then you may have hemorrhoids. If this is the case then there are instructions for that in the "*Third Trimester section*".

If you are breast-feeding, your milk should come in at about 48 hours after the birth of your baby. See '*Breast issues*' section for information on this. By this time, you should have had plenty of rest and be up walking around without concerns. You should move with ease and feel like doing many routine activities. Caution: There is still an open wound where the placenta detached itself from the uterine wall, do not pick up anything over 20 pounds and do not stand for over two hours without sitting or laying to rest for a few minutes (longer if necessary).

Within 24 - 48 hours after you feel up to getting around it should be okay for you to go with someone for a short walk, maybe down the street a ways to get a little fresh air. Do not overdo. If this activity increases your blood flow, then you still need to take it easy for a few more days.

Mother's deserve to be mothered for a couple of weeks after giving birth. Take care of you. Having two weeks of meals prepared in the freezer before you give birth will help give you a chance to have wholesome food without the effort of cooking during your recovery.

No illness or disease is normal after childbirth. If you get sick, weak, or depressed it is not normal and there are solutions. You have enough information in your hands to do something more than just lay there and be a victim. Be proactive.

How long to wait before having sex? This is a question that is more frequently asked by our ladies than by their husbands. The fact is that women are all different and depending on how well the birth went, there are different degrees of damage that may have taken place during the birth. If there were tears or an episiotomy then it will take longer than if it was a smooth, natural process where there was no damage to the birth canal, perineum, or cervix. If there was a tear, or an episiotomy, then enough time needs to be given to allow those areas to heal. There is always the open site where the placenta was attached to the uterine wall. This needs to heal. It is important to give your body a chance to heal properly before any kind of sexual activity.

As long as there is bleeding then there is something that is not, yet, healed. Sexual activity can increase the chances of infection getting into the open wounds. Sex can also open up areas that are sutured. The sutures are there for a reason. There are muscles that go from the inside of the hip down to the pelvic floor (perineum) to hold the hips into place. Women who have tears that are not allowed to heal properly have a much higher chance of having long term low back and pelvic pain than other women. Allow that pelvic floor to heal.

I approve clients to resume sexual activity as soon as 1) There has been no bleeding for 48 hours or more. 2) She feels up to it <u>and</u> there is no pain involved. 3) There is no odor of infection or any other discharge. When all of these are good then I give the go ahead; but never before that.

The first few times back to love making it is good to use warm olive oil, as a lubricant, to help heal and restore the natural elasticity to the muscles. It also is important to take it very slow and easy as to not cause any damage. If there is any pain, then stop immediately.

If he hit's the cervix, (it will be very tender-like he is going too deep), then it shows that the cervix has not healed yet and could be dropped down. It would be good to give it another week or so. If you could do some crunches, or setups, then it would help to pull that cervix back up to where it belongs and it will not interfere with sex. The best way to do this is to do as many as you can without pain and then stop, even if that is only one or two. Wait three or four days and, again, do as many as you can without pain. Generally, you can do two or three times as many the second session as you did the first because time was given to heal. Every part of the body is healed through diet and rest. It is opened up to be healed with exercise and day to day life. So the pattern is to exercise one day, then eat properly and rest in between exercise sessions, then exercise again in three or four days. If bleeding increases during exercise then your body is not ready for it yet and it is causing damage.

Once your body has had a chance to heal then try again. Most of our ladies are able to resume an active sex life within two to four weeks after giving birth. However, rarely does one of our ladies have severe damage with her birth. Those conditions would be expected to take another two to four weeks to heal.

Notes_____

~26~
My Powerfully Pregnant Journal

My last menstrual cycle started _____

The date of conception was _____

Estimated due date is _____

Special notes up to date _____

_____

_____

_____

_____

When I realized I was pregnant _____

_____

_____

_____

_____

My pregnancy was confirmed by _____

The first person I told was _____

The first sign of pregnancy was _____

_____

This is the _____ child. (1st, 2nd, 3rd etc)

I am excited about the birth of this child because _____

_____

_____

_____

_____

The Hopes and Dreams I have for My Child are _____

_____
_____
_____
_____
_____
_____

Special things I have planned for me during this pregnancy _____

_____
_____
_____

Things family has done to help welcome this new little addition _____

_____
_____
_____
_____

Symptoms I experienced during previous pregnancies that I wish to avoid during this pregnancy. _____

_____
_____
_____

Did we get a sneak-peek at baby with an ultrasound? _____

_____
_____
_____
_____

Other notes

First Trimester!

First Trimester expectations _____

_____
_____
_____
_____

Symptoms I have experienced during the first trimester _____

_____
_____
_____
_____
_____
_____
_____
_____
_____

Positive outcomes I have had from a simple change of diet _____

_____
_____
_____
_____
_____
_____
_____

Supplements that made me feel better _____

_____
_____
_____
_____

Ooops! Signs I get from eating the wrong foods _____

_____
_____
_____
_____

What I am doing to resolve first trimester discomforts or problems _____

_____
_____
_____
_____
_____
_____
_____
_____
_____
_____
_____

First trimester successes!!

Special people who have supported my approach to my pregnancy

Trips, special occasions and experiences that have happened during this first trimester

The happiest day of my first trimester was

Specific things I am doing for a better labor and delivery experience

Checkup notes

Powerfully Pregnant

Second Trimester!!

Second Trimester expectations _____

_____

_____

_____

Plans I have for the second trimester _____

_____

_____

_____

Symptoms I have experienced during my second trimester _____

_____

_____

_____

_____

_____

Positive outcomes I have had from a simple change of diet or supplements

_____

_____

_____

_____

_____

My favorite supplements are _____

_____
_____
_____
_____
_____

Mistakes made and learned from! _____

_____
_____
_____
_____

What I am doing to resolve second trimester discomforts or problems

_____
_____
_____
_____
_____
_____
_____
_____
_____
_____
_____

Second trimester successes!!

Special people who have supported me during my pregnancy

Special occasions and experiences that have happened during the second trimester

The happiest day of my second trimester was _____

_____
_____
_____
_____

Moments that made me feel the most happy about my pregnancy

_____
_____
_____
_____
_____
_____
_____
_____

The best recipe I got this trimester was _____

_____
_____
_____

Specific things I am now doing for a better labor and delivery experience

_____
_____
_____
_____
_____
_____
_____

Some of the wonderful things that I would like this baby to know are

_____
_____
_____
_____
_____
_____
_____

Checkup notes _____

_____
_____
_____
_____
_____
_____
_____
_____
_____
_____
_____
_____
_____

Third Trimester!!!

Ways I have taken on personal responsibility to make this pregnancy better are _____

How has this pregnancy been different than others, for myself, friends or family members? _____

I intend to make my baby feel loved by _____

Possible names being considered

Checkup notes

Powerfully Pregnant

The Birth!!!!

First signs of labor _____
_____
_____
_____
_____
_____

About Labor and Delivery _____
_____
_____
_____
_____
_____
_____
_____
_____
_____
_____
_____

Birth took place at _____
Address _____
_____

Primary Birth Attendant _____
Assistant Birth Attendant _____

Powerfully Pregnant

About Baby

Sweet Little (Name) _____ *was born*

To (Parents Name) _____

on (Date) _____

At (Time) _____

Cute as can be at ____ *inches in Length and Weighing* _____

Eyes _____

Hair _____

Place picture here!

Recipes

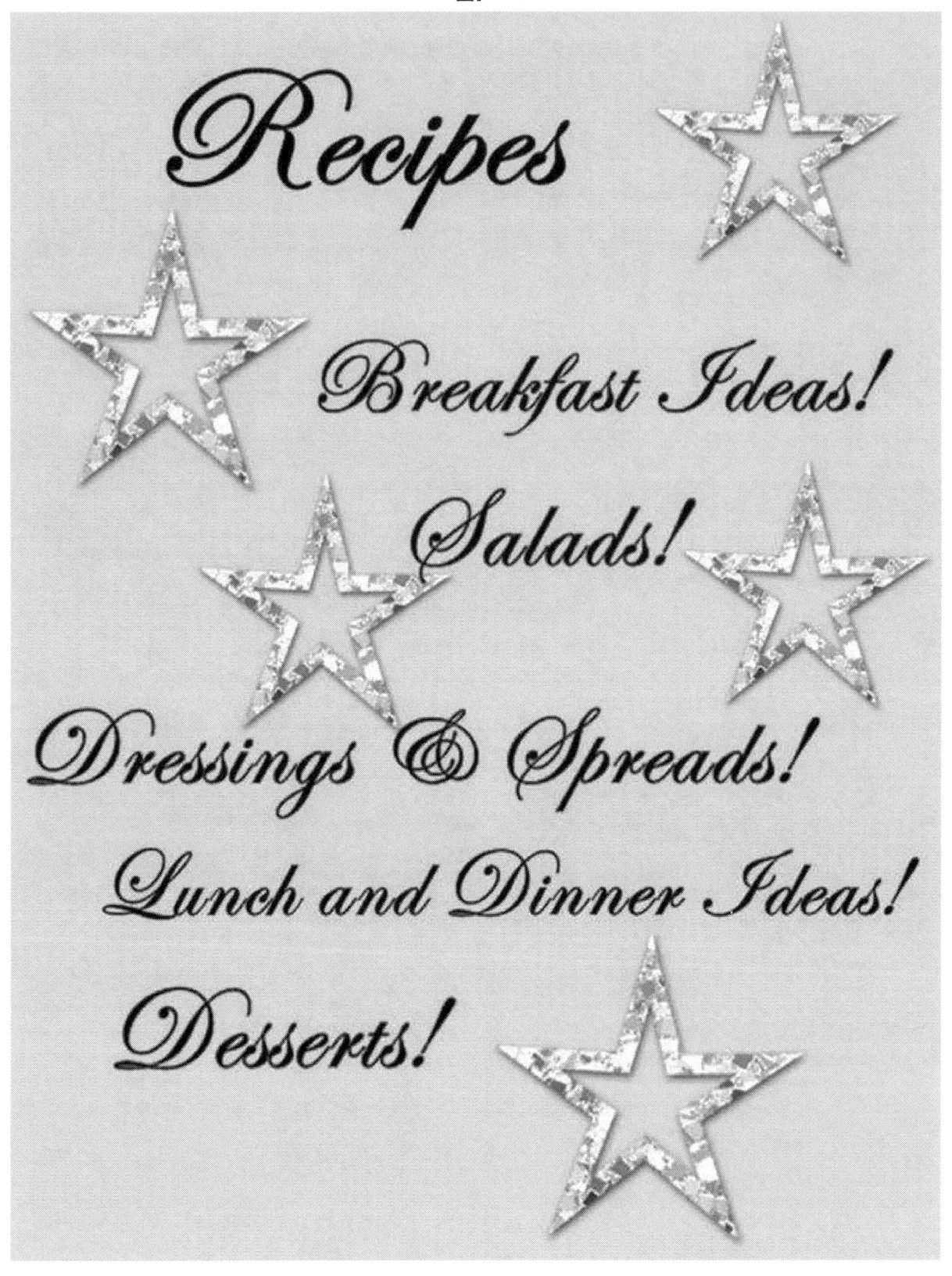

Breakfast Ideas!

Salads!

Dressings & Spreads!

Lunch and Dinner Ideas!

Desserts!

The hardest part of the program, most will agree, is finding what is acceptable to eat. For that reason we decided to include a recipe section to assist your efforts. Recipes have been donated by those who have been on this diet and found positive results with it. This is also the reason some are formatted a little differently than others, everyone has their own way of explaining things. These were some of the recipes they felt you would enjoy and their name appears with the recipe. This may or may not mean they originated the recipe, it means it is who donated it to us and we are recognizing them and their efforts to help others. A warm 'Thank you' to each.

Tweaking (which means to fine tune or adjust) recipes is a term we use for altering a recipe to fit into our diet. Around our house we will look through recipe books and see what looks good then we tear it apart and see what we can do to make it fit our way of life. Fact is, we don't miss out on much.

If a recipe calls for sugar, we play with it to see how it works with stevia, honey, agave nectar etc. If it calls for flour, we play with the same basic principle with rolled oats or other whole grain cereal or maybe almond butter, etc. If it calls for cayenne we tone it down with either mild chili powder or else sweet peppers. If it calls for tomatoes we have found we can substitute applesauce or maybe mashed sweet potatoes instead, depending on the recipe. We play with different things and found there are a ka-zillion ways to make things work. We just have to think beyond the usual boundaries or limitations. The possibilities are endless and we are never deprived. Below (between the stars) is an example of a 'barbeque sauce' we tweaked... because we did not want the negative affects that may feed problems like acid reflux, arthritis, heartburn or colic in baby that could occur from the original recipe.
****
For educational reasons, we are putting the original recipe here so you can see how it was as altered. This one does not fit diet.

Barbeque Sauce
2 Tbsp Butter
1 large Onion, diced
2 cloves Garlic, minced
16 oz Tomato sauce
2/3 C Apple Cider Vinegar
2/3 C Brown sugar
1 Tbsp prepared Mustard
2 Tbsp Cayenne
1 tsp Black Pepper

Barbeque Sauce (revised)
(Donna Young)
2 Tbsp Olive oil
1 large Onion, diced
2 cloves Garlic, minced
8 oz Applesauce, unsweetened
8 oz mashed Sweet Potatoes
2/3 C Apple Cider Vinegar
2/3 C Honey
1 Tbsp prepared Mustard
2 tsp mild Chili Powder
½ tsp Black Pepper

Lightly sauté the onion an garlic in the olive oil. Add in applesauce, sweet potatoes, honey, vinegar, mustard, chili powder and pepper. Bring to a boil, stir and cook just until the mustard is dissolved together with the rest of the ingredients. Use on all kinds of meats, omelets, eggs, veggies.
****

~~~~~BREAKFAST IDEAS~~~~~

Holt's Banana Cherry Smoothie
(Holt Young)

2 cups Almond Milk
1 cup Cherries (frozen or fresh, pitted)
1 large Banana
2 cups ice cubes
8 drops Vanilla Crème Stevia
8 drops English Toffee Stevia

Blend together in blender until smooth. Drink immediately.

Banana Nut Muffins
(Brooke Sprouse)

5 C Rolled oats
2 C Water
1 tsp Real Sat
3 Tbsp baking powder
¾ C Honey
¼ C Olive Oil
3 Eggs
1 tsp Vanilla
¼ tsp Cardamom
¼ tsp Nutmeg
3 very ripe Bananas, mashed
3 small Apples, peeled and diced
2 cups Nuts, chopped

Mix together in order listed. Reserve ½ of the nuts to sprinkle on top. Fill muffin tins lined with paper muffin cups. Sprinkle with remaining nuts. Bake at 350' until golden and set (about 40-50 min)

Blueberry Bread
(Elizabeth Bailey)

5 Cups Rolled Oats
2 Cups water
1 tsp Real Salt
3 Tbsp Baking Powder
¾ Cup Honey
¼ Cup Olive Oil
3 Eggs
1 Pint Fresh Blueberries
1 tsp. Vanilla
¼ tsp Cardamom
¼ tsp Nutmeg

Bake in oiled loaf pan at 350' until golden and set.

Pancakes
(Elizabeth Bailey)

15 Cups raw Rolled Oats
8 Cups Almond or Rice Milk
10 beaten eggs
8 tsp. Vanilla
1 tsp Real Salt
4 Tbsp Baking Powder
Cardamom
Nutmeg
Stir thoroughly,
Go ahead and add frozen blueberries if you wish!!
Cook on an oiled griddle as any pancake and serve with Agave Nectar, Maple Syrup or any fruit sweetened with Honey.

Banana pancakes: Omit blueberries, cardamom and nutmeg. Add 3 mashed bananas and 1 ½ tsp cinnamon.

Breakfast Casserole
(Elizabeth Bailey)

4 lbs cooked Turkey Sausage
2 dozen beaten eggs
2 large bags fresh or frozen spinach
  or
1 bag Broccoli Slaw
3 Tbsp. Prepared Specialty Mustard
Real Salt
Rosemary
Chopped onion
Garlic
Onion powder
*Optional--sliced mushrooms
Top with garlic chives
Bake at 350' till set.

Cherry Smoothie
(Melissa Morgan)

1 ½ cups frozen Cherries
1 Banana
1 cup fresh spinach
½ cup Rolled Oats
1/8 - ¼ cup Agave
5-10 Almonds (optional)
1 cup Rice or Almond Milk

Add all ingredients and blend. If you like, add peeled apple or change fruits around to your liking. Sometimes I'll add frozen juice concentrate or honey in place of agave.

Doug's Breakfast Smoothie
(Tracy Slack)

2 Cups fresh spinach or mild tasting lettuce
1-2 Cups berries
1 Banana
Rice milk to desired thickness
5 drops Berry flavored Stevia
Optional: Free range eggs, whey protein, kelp, alfalfa etc.
(Our 5 year old loves this drink! We do, too!)

Raw Granola
(Revised by Tracy Slack)

3 C Organic Rolled Oats
1 ½ C chopped Pecans
¼ C raw Sunflower, raw Pumpkin seeds or Pine nuts (shelled)
¼ C raw Sesame Seeds
1 C chopped dried Dates
¼ C golden Raisins or dry Cranberries
¼ C cut up, dried Apricots
¼ C Acacia fiber (or ground wheat germ, wheat bran or ground flax seed.
About 3-4 Tbsp raw local Honey

Mix dry ingredients. Add honey until oats start to "roll". Do not want too sticky. Add rice milk and enjoy!!
 All ingredients would normally keep in the pantry. Mixed together they will still keep in the pantry.
 If you use pure maple syrup or agave nectar instead of honey then mixture will need to be refrigerated.

Moist Granola Bars
(Elizabeth Bailey)

Mix:
1 ½ cups Dried fruits
2 Tbsp Molasses
4 Tbsp Olive oil
6 Eggs
1 cup Honey
1 tsp Vanilla

Mix:
3 cups Puffed Cereal (wheat or Rice)
3 ½ cups rolled oats
2 tsp. Carob powder
1 ½ tsp Bee Pollen
½ tsp Kelp granules or Real Salt
2 tsp Cinnamon

Combine mixes and press into an 8 inch glass baking dish. Bake at 350F until golden. Cut into squares and store.

French Toast
(Elizabeth Bailey)

Dip thick Batter Bread slices into a mix of:
Scrambled raw eggs
Rice milk
Orange flavoring
Nutmeg
Vanilla extract
Cook each side on olive oiled griddle till golden brown.
Serve with pure maple syrup or agave.

Pumpkin Pancakes
(Elizabeth Bailey)

1 large can pumpkin puree
¼ tsp Real Salt
2 tsp Baking powder
4 Eggs
2 ½ cups raw rolled oats
3 ½ tsp Pumpkin pie spice
2 tsp. Green Stevia plant powder
Mix well and cook as pancakes on griddle.

Holiday Smoothie
(Holt Young)

1 cup fresh Cranberry sauce
2 ½ cups Almond Milk
2 Tbsp Honey or Agave
1 tray Ice cubes
1 tsp Vanilla extract
Blend together and serve immediately.

Tracy's Granola
(Tracy Slack)

4 Cups Rolled Oats
½ Cup Wheat Germ (unsweetened)
½ Cup Sesame Seeds
5 Cups Nuts and Seeds, raw, shelled and unsalted (Soak overnight and dry prior to use for additional nutritional value) I use 1 Cup each of my favorites: Sunflower seeds, Cashews, Pumpkin seeds, Pine Nuts and Pecans.
1 Cup Chipped Coconut
1 Cup Dried Fruit (I use ¼ Cup quantities of my favorites diced Apricot, Cranberries, Dates and Raisins.
¾ Cup Honey
2/3 Cup Olive or Coconut Oil

Combine rolled oats, wheat germ, nuts and seeds. Combine honey and oil and stir into dry ingredients. Stir in dried fruit. Bake at 300 degrees for 40-45 minutes in 13"X9" pan. Stir every 15 minutes. Stir while cooling to prevent clumping.

Nancy's (Mom's) Granola
(Tracy Slack)

4 Cups Rolled Oats
1 Cups Shredded Coconut
1 Cup Sunflower seeds
½ Wheat Germ (unsweetened)
1 Cup Pumpkin seeds
1 Cup Cashews
1 Cup Almonds
1 Cup Walnuts
½ Cup Sesame Seeds
¾ Cup honey
2/3 Cup Light Olive oil
1 cup Raisins or ½ Cup dried Cranberries

Mix honey and oil and set aside. Combine remaining ingredients (except raisins / cranberries) and stir. Pour honey and oil over dry ingredients. Pour into 9X13" baking pan and bake at 300 degrees for 40-45 minutes. Stir every 10-15 minutes! Then add raisins. Stir while cooling to prevent clumping.

Breakfast Buffet
(Wendy Ray)

Most winter mornings, our breakfast consists of one of several hot cereals with various nuts, seeds and fruit. But on busy summer mornings at our house, we're up with the sun, working in the garden or trying to get a few chores or school assignments going, so no one wants to spend much time in the kitchen.

Lately, our favorite instant breakfast is a raw oat buffet (we use other rolled grains when we have them -wheat, amaranth, barley- the ideal would be to have our own roller and roll a variety of fresh grains every day).

Buffet items include:
Carob powder (sweet enough that no additional sweetener is needed - the kids especially love chunks of carob powder: they are like chocolate chips swimming around in their almond milk)
Diced apples, bananas and other fruit (frozen berries, raisins, fresh pineapple... whatever we have on hand)
Dried coconut (the kind that isn't covered in sugar)
Sunflower seeds
Ground flax seeds
Cinnamon
Juice concentrate or honey to sweeten if needed
Sometimes I have a pan of water simmering on the stove, in case anyone is in the mood for hot cereal; they just add water to their own bowl. :)
On birthdays and other special occasions, we might add plain yogurt too; or a banana-strawberry smoothie.

Everyone's favorite is oats, carob, a dash of salt, sliced bananas, raisins and almond milk. Quick "chocolate pudding" effect.
These days, this idea beats homemade granola. Hands down.
If you're considering trying this, start with plenty of variety and make it pretty, like a real buffet. ;)

Powerfully Pregnant

Healthy Morning Glory Muffins
(Tabitha Newman)

Ingredients
2 1/2 cups rolled oats
2 T. Corn Starch
3/4 C. Honey
2 T. Molasses
3 teaspoons ground cinnamon
2 teaspoons baking soda
1/2 teaspoon salt
3 eggs
3/4 cup applesauce (unsweetened)
1/2 cup olive oil
1 teaspoon vanilla extract
2 cups grated carrots
1 medium tart apple, peeled and grated
1 (8 ounce) can crushed pineapple, drained (unsweetened)
1/2 cup flaked coconut, (unsweetened)
1/2 cup raisins (optional)
1/2 cup chopped walnuts (optional)

Directions

1. In a large bowl, combine the rolled oats, corn starch, cinnamon, soda, and salt. In another bowl, combine the honey, molasses, eggs, applesauce, oil and vanilla. Stir in carrots, apple, pineapple, coconut, raisins and nuts.

2. Fill greased or paper-lined muffin cups two-thirds full. Bake at 350 degrees F for 20-24 minutes or until a toothpick comes out clean. Cool for 5 minutes before removing from pans to wire racks.

Pumpkin Cake
(Tabitha Newman)

1 c pumpkin puree
1 c almond butter
1/2 c raw honey
2 eggs
1 ½ t baking powder
½ t baking soda
1 t vanilla extract
1 t cinnamon
¼ t nutmeg
¼ t cloves

Preheat your oven to 350F. In a medium sized bowl, combine all the cake ingredients and mix thoroughly to combine. Pour into an 8×8 oven safe baking dish. Bake until completely cooked through, about 30 minutes.

Sherie and I love this recipe and it gives you something to supplement all of those sweets around the Thanksgiving table. (DY: Great anytime day or night and healthy!)

Hot Cereal Variations
(Tracy Slack)

7 Grain Cereal (I like the wheat free)
1 Cup Water
½ Cup 7 Grain Cereal
Pinch Real Salt
In saucepan, mix together and bring to a boil over medium heat.
Once boiling, cook minutes.
Add salt.
Add any of these variations.
Cut up dates, raisins, and dried cranberries.
Add walnuts in big pieces, break by hand.
Add maple Syrup to taste.

Cream of Wheat:
1 Cup Water
1/3 Cup Cream of Wheat
Pinch of Real Salt
Bring water to boil then add cereal and cook for 3 minutes. Add salt.
Add any of the following:
Dried raspberries
Broken Walnuts
Local Honey to taste

Steel Cut Oats (aka Irish or Scottish Oats):
1 Cup Water
½ Cup Steel Cut Oats
Pinch Real Salt

Place water and oats in pan. Bring to a boil. Turn down heat and boil mixture for 7 minutes. Add salt.

Add any of the following:
Broken Pecans
Golden Raisins
Pure Maple Syrup to taste

Turkey Sausage
(Tracy Slack)

1 ½ Tbsp Real salt
1/8 tsp Pepper
1 tsp dried Sage
1 tsp pure Maple Syrup
1 tsp finely chopped Garlic
1 lb ground Turkey meat.
Buy ground turkey and put into a skillet with the rest of seasonings. This replaces pork sausage for breakfast.

Fruit on Sweet Brown Rice with Coconut Milk
(Tracy Slack)

1 C cooked Sweet Brown short grain Rice (We like the Lundberg brand) into a bowl In a separate bowl, mix 1 cup Coconut Milk with 2 Tbls Honey (or other natural sweetener) and 2 pinches Real salt. Pour liquid mixture atop rice. Place 1 fresh fruit, peeled and diced (we use pear, peach, or whatever fruit is really ripe and sweet) Note: Best served warm. If your coconut milk has been refrigerated, warm it on the stove first (coconut milk will curdle if boiled!) A traditional summer recipe but a favorite a dessert at our house anytime of the year.

Hash
(Elizabeth Bailey)

Small amount of olive oil in medium heat skillet. Add thin sliced sweet potatoes and cook till tender. Add Real salt, pepper and thyme to taste. Add diced, cooked turkey or beef and chopped onion. Heat through and add chopped tomatillos and fresh spinach and a little basil. Heat through and serve topped with eggs.

Turkey Sausage Gravy
(Tracy Slack)

1 lb Turkey Sausage
1 Onion, finely chopped
1 green, Bell pepper, chopped (opt)
2 Tbsp Garlic, minced
Real salt and pepper to taste
1 tsp minced fresh Sage
1 tsp minced fresh Thyme
Olive oil to cook above with 2 C Rice milk (or coconut milk--it's thicker and richer-- also sweeter, so may want to leave out maple syrup in sausage)
2 tsp Chicken bouillon (I like McCormick's chicken paste w/o MSG)
¼ C minced fresh Parsley

1. In a skillet, on medium heat, cook sausage, onion, garlic, salt, pepper, sage and thyme. Cook until turkey is crumbly.
2. Stir in Rice milk and incorporate well. Add chicken bouillon. Thicken mixture with thickener of choice (corn starch, tapioca starch or arrowroot). If it thickens too much, add more rice milk.
3. Just before serving, add parsley.

Sweet Italian Sausage
(Donna Young)

2 lb Ground Turkey
1 Tbsp Real salt
1 Tbsp ground Fennel seed (if grinding your own, do not over grind)
1 ½ Tbsp sweet Paprika
1 Tbsp finely minced fresh Garlic
1 Tbsp Honey
1 tsp Black Pepper
3 Tbsp Red Wine Vinegar
Mix all the seasonings together then pour over the ground turkey and mix well. You can use this recipe right away but it gets better after about 12 hours in the fridge.

Omelets
(Donna Young)

Omelets are a wholesome high protein breakfast. Almost anything you could have put in a sandwich can be put in an omelet. Leftovers make great ones, too! Some of our favorite fillings/toppings are listed here:

Browned hamburger, onion, bell pepper and cheese.
Left over White Bean and Chicken Chili.
Cheese and Barbecue sauce
Left over roast and veggies
Turkey and maple-pecan sweet potatoes.
Confetti Salad.
Beans, cheese, onions and peppers.
Refried beans, green chili peppers, onions and browned ground meat.
Sweet Italian Turkey Sausage and onions topped with Turkey Sausage gravy.
Dill Chicken, Dill pickles and onion.
Asian Chicken and veggies.
Rebecca's Nachos.

Bear came up with this wonderful idea: Make the omelets 'open faced' to get more toppings in them... ..like a tostada!

Notes

Powerfully Pregnant

~~~~~LUNCH AND DINNER IDEAS~~~~~

Barbecued Burgers
(Donna Young)

1 lb lean Ground Turkey or Beef
½ C chopped Onion
1 Egg
½ tsp Garlic salt
2 tsp Worcestershire sauce
About 1 cup Rolled Oats.

Mix ground meat, onion and egg together then add in enough rolled oats to form into patties. Bake or grill as desired. Remember that it is recommended that all meat b e completely cooked to kill any bacteria etc. During the last five minutes of cooking we put on a barbecue sauce made from the next recipe then add extra sauce on the plate.

Barbecue Sauce
(Donna Young)

2 Tbsp Olive oil
1 large Onion, diced
2 cloves Garlic, minced
8 oz Applesauce, unsweetened
8 oz mashed Sweet Potatoes
2/3 C Apple Cider Vinegar
2/3 C Honey
1 Tbsp prepared Mustard
2 tsp mild Chili Powder
½ tsp Black Pepper

Lightly sauté the onion an garlic in the olive oil. Add in applesauce, sweet potatoes, honey, vinegar, mustard, chili powder and pepper. Bring to a boil and cook just until the mustard is dissolved together with the rest of the ingredients. Use on all kinds of meats, omelets, eggs, veggies.

Note: Can be eaten hot or cold. Put the leftovers in a jar in the fridge… they are used in a little while for things like eggs, meats, veggies etc.

Dill Chicken
(Edelweiss Oberhansley)

2 Tbsp Olive Oil
2 Tbsp Lemon juice
1 tsp Real Salt
½ tsp Garlic Powder
Dash of Black Pepper
½ tsp Paprika
1 Tbsp Dill weed (Dill leaves)
6 Large Chicken thighs (or 8 small)

Coat skillet with Olive Oil. Mix the spices together with Lemon juice and pour into skillet. Bring to a boil and put chicken into pan with mix. Cover and cook on medium heat for 15 minutes.
Turn chicken over, replace lid and turn down heat a little to Medium Low. Cook until completely done, turning as needed. Serve with Wild rice and vegetable of your choice. Enjoy!!

Summer Italian Chicken
(Elizabeth Bailey)

Cook 6 lbs Chicken Breasts
(boned and skinned) in Olive oil until golden brown.
Stir in:
Chopped zucchini and / or
Yellow Summer Squash
Chopped Onion
Garlic
Greens (frozen spinach, fresh collards are the best
Mushrooms
Real Salt to taste
Oregano
Basil
Parsley
Cook until veggies are al dente.
Serve over rice or spaghetti squash.

*May add green or yellow fresh garden tomatoes as available IF no high acid conditions are a concern.

Herbed Chicken
(Elizabeth Bailey)

Bake:
6 lbs boneless, skinless Chicken
Olive Oil
2 Tbsp minced, dry Onion
3 cloves Garlic
2 tsp Thyme
1 tsp. Real Salt
1 tsp. Black Pepper
½ tsp Rosemary
½ tsp Sage

Deviled Eggs
(Rebecca Dimick)

5 boiled Eggs
½ tsp Mustard
1/8 tsp Vinegar
2 Tbl Miracle Whip (or Blender Mayo)
½ tsp Sweet Relish
1 tsp chopped Onion
1 tsp chopped Pepper
Dash of Salt
Dash of Pepper
Paprika

Directions:
1. Shell eggs. Take yolks out.
2. Mix egg yolks with other ingredients.
3. Spoon mixture into egg whites.
4. Serve.

Powerfully Pregnant

Steamed Dinners
(Donna Young)

The first time I was introduced to steamed food, I thought "What? Steamed chicken? You have got to be kidding!" But one bite and I was sold. The meat is thoroughly cooked, moist and tender. Good stuff!

When Holt and I travel, we always take the steamer with us. We can make up fast, healthy meals for two without any real effort or mess. Everything tastes wonderful. Holt can cook dinner for us when traveling and she loves it! Far better than eating café food. She likes to create tasty, healthy food.

First we put in the cleaned meat and carrots. Put a little seasoning on the chicken. Turn on the steamer. After the meat and carrots have steamed for about a half hour we put the second shelf on that has the washed corn and cauliflower.

Then, just as everything is about finished (in about 20 minutes) we add the sugar snap peas. We like those just warmed through and still crunchy. Dinner is finished in about an hour. A salad on the side, fruit for dessert... . We are happy and healthy.

There are several companies that make food steamers and we have had different brands. We are very happy with all of them. Some are a little larger and we are able to cook for 3-4 as opposed to 2. All the foods taste fresher and healthier. We have had beef, turkey, fish and lots of different kinds of vegetables steamed! We never feel deprived.

Flaming Gorge Trout
(Melissa Morgan)

We thawed the fish and washed it. Beat some eggs and dipped the fish in the egg. We then dipped the fish in walnuts that I had chopped in the blender. I salted and peppered them and fried in olive oil. I'm sure it would have been fine to bake it also. Pretty tasty, I must say!

Acorn Squash
(Elizabeth Bailey)

Half and Seed the Squash
In a baking dish with 1-2" water put squash, cut side up. Fill halves with diced apple and maple syrup, sprinkle with pumpkin pie spice and a dot with butter. Bake at 350' until tender.

Apricot Chicken
(Elizabeth Bailey)

6lbs boneless, skinless Chicken Breasts cooked in olive oil
1 large onion, chopped
Real Salt and Pepper, to taste
Mix together to taste:
1 Cup Apricot Jam
Parsley
Ginger root powder
Pour over chicken and cook until flavors absorb into chicken, about 15 minutes on med-low heat.

Asian Chicken Dinner
(Elizabeth Bailey)

6 lbs boneless, skinless Chicken Breasts cooked in a little Olive Oil, Balsamic Vinegar, Honey, Ginger Root powder, Cornstarch to thicken. Stir in Stir Fry veggies and serve with steamed Rice. Top with chopped, raw Nuts

Honey Mustard Chicken
(Elizabeth Bailey)

Cook 6lbs. Boneless skinless Chicken in Olive Oil
Add:
Brown Mustard
Honey
Garlic powder
Real Salt
Simmer 10 minutes, stirring often.

Chicken Soup
(Elizabeth Bailey)

Boil Chicken or Turkey carcasses by covering with water and boiling down by at least 1/3
Then add:
Cooked Chicken
Carrots, sliced
Celery, sliced
Onion, diced
Real Salt to taste
Pepper
Bay leaf
Boil till veggies are done.

Basil Burgers
(Elizabeth Bailey)

Mix together:
6 lbs ground Turkey
¾ cup jarred minced Garlic
Way too much Worcestershire sauce
Scant ¼ c. dried Basil
Form into patties and fry or bake.

Beef Ribs
(Elizabeth Bailey)

Mix:
Molasses
Real Salt
Vinegar
Chili powder, mild
Black Pepper
Old Bay
Thyme
Onion powder
Honey
Garlic
Pour over ribs. Cover with foil and bake at low heat until meat falls off the bone.

Sloppy Joes
(Elizabeth Bailey)

In large skillet brown 6lb Ground meat (Beef or Turkey)
Then add:
Real Salt and pepper to taste
2 Onions, chopped
3 cloves Garlic, chopped
3 Carrots, grated
3 Celery ribs, chopped
1 bell pepper, chopped
6 Tbsp Honey
6 Tbsp vinegar
Worcestershire sauce
2 cups Chicken stock
Cook through. Serve over Batter Bread toast with pickles.

Hamburger Soup
(Rebecca Dimick)

1 Lb Ground Beef
1 chopped Onion
1 can Green Beans
6 small Potatoes
1 can Whole Kernel Corn
1 can Cream of Mushroom Soup
4-6 cups Water
 Directions:
1. Brown ground beef
2. Drain fat and add onion
3. Put in large pot with green beans, corn, potato, mushroom soup and water.
4. Cook until done through.

Spaghetti-less Meat Dish
(Elizabeth Bailey)

Cook in skillet:
6 lbs ground Turkey
Garlic
2 chopped Onions
2 jars roasted Red Bell Peppers
Frozen Corn
Chopped Mushrooms
Spinach or Collard Greens (Fresh, frozen or canned)
Basil
Oregano
Real Salt
Serve over cooked rice or spaghetti squash.

Beef Stew
(Holt Young)

1 lb Ground Beef, browned, drained
1 Onion diced
1 cup Frozen Corn
4 Carrots, peeled, cut
2 Cloves Garlic, minced
Mix together in stew pan, cover with water plus one more inch. Add seasonings of choice (I like Sloppy Joe or Spaghetti spices)
Boil for 20 minutes and add:
½ head of Cabbage, shredded
10 Radishes, cut in fourths
Cook for an additional 5 minutes and serve.

Salisbury Steaks
(Elizabeth Bailey)

Mix together:
Ground meat
Worcestershire sauce
Onion, chopped
Egg, beaten
Real Salt
Parsley
Once mixed, add enough Rolled oats to get it to hold together for patties. Shape into patties, fry or bake until cooked through and top with gravy made of:
Beef stock
Olive oil
Worcestershire sauce
Onions, chopped
Garlic, chopped
Cornstarch to thicken when boiled.

Turkey Sausage Meatballs
(Elizabeth Bailey)

Mix:
Ground Turkey
Rosemary
Garlic, chopped
Fennel seeds
Eggs
Real Salt
Enough rolled oats to get mixture to hold shape. Shape into balls. Then put on olive oiled baking sheet and bake at 400F until cooked through turning once. (Depending on size of meatball, about 30 minutes total with 15 minutes on each side)

Cooked carrots
~No you don't boil them!~
(Elizabeth Bailey)

Wash and chop Carrots into bite size chunks. Put them into a lidded cast iron pot and drizzle with Olive oil. Bake at 350'. May stir several times to caramelize more of the carrots. They are best when brown and moist, not dry or charred.

Cheating Chili--not the real deal
(Elizabeth Bailey)

Red, Black and White dry Beans
Water
Cooked, ground Turkey
Onions, chopped
Garlic powder
Real Salt
Paprika
Oregano
Chili Powder (Mild)
Slow cook adding water as needed till beans are soft and a thick sauce is formed.

Chinese Meatball Soup
(Bear Hunter)

1 lb Ground Beef
¾ cup Rolled Oats
2 Tbsp Soy Sauce
1 ½ tsp Ginger
½ tsp Black Pepper
¼ cup Chicken Broth
1 Egg
(optional diced Sweet Peppers)
Soup
14-16 ounces Chicken broth
1 cup Water
1 pkg fresh Snow Peas
½ small head of shredded Cabbage
½ cup chopped Onion
1 clove Garlic, minced

Prepare meatballs: Stir ingredients together, shape into 1 ¼ inch balls and place on slightly oiled (olive) broiler pan. Bake at 400' for 15-20 minutes.

Heat chicken broth, water and garlic to a boil. Add in onions let cook a few minutes then add in cabbage, peas and meatballs. Let veggies heat through but do not over cook. Peas and cabbage should remain firm. Serve hot.

Variations: Use Chicken, instead of meatballs. Use celery, water chestnuts, turnips, thinly sliced carrots etc. Most vegetable are going to be good in this one!!

White Bean & Chicken Chili
(Melissa Mittanck)

8 oz shredded Chicken
1 Cup chopped Onion
1 chopped pepper (green, red or yellow)
1- 4.5 oz. can chopped green chilies
2 tsp Ground Cumin
½ tsp dried Oregano
3 ½ Cups Chicken Broth
3 cans White Northern Beans
2 Garlic cloves
Add everything to the crock pot and cook 8-10 hours in low or 4-5 hours on high.

White Bean and Chicken Chili
(Rebecca Dimick)

4 raw Chicken Breasts, cubed
4 crushed, fresh garlic cloves
1 cup chopped onion
2 cans White Beans, drained
2-4 cups Chicken Broth
¼ cup chopped, fresh Cilantro
1tsp Paprika
½ tsp Real Salt
1 tsp black pepper
½ Cup low acid tomatoes
Fresh Avocado, sliced

In large pot heat 1 Tbsp Olive oil. Cook chicken breasts, garlic and onion on medium heat for 5-10 minutes, stirring frequently. When chicken is cooked, add beans and enough broth to bring to desired consistency, paprika, salt and pepper. Cook for 10 minutes. Serve and top with tomatoes, fresh cilantro and avocado.

Chicken, Bean & Rice Soup
(Rebecca Dimick)

2 Cups cooked or canned Chicken
2 Cups cooked Brown Rice
1 Can Black Beans
1- 1 ½ Quarts Water
2 Cups slice Zucchini
1 Cup Broccoli, chopped
1 Cup Celery, chopped
½ Cup Whole Cherry Tomatoes
1 tsp Garlic Salt and Black Pepper
2 tsp Basil
Dash turmeric
2 Tbsp fresh Cilantro

In large pot, combine all ingredients except for cilantro. Let boil 1-2 minutes, then put a lid on it and reduce heat to low / medium low and let cook 10-15 minutes or until broccoli and zucchini are tender. Add cilantro and serve.

Thai Chicken and Asparagus Soup
(Tracy Slack)

12 oz cooked and pieced Chicken
1 can Coconut Milk
1 cup Rice milk
2 Tbsp Fish Sauce (Rufina Patis Thia brand has no MSG)
1 Tbsp dried Basil leaves or about 10 fresh basil leaves
2 Tbsp minced Ginger
8 oz Fresh Asparagus, chopped thin or diced
8 oz fresh or dried Mushrooms (optional)

Cook asparagus. Saute veggies w/ seasonings. Add other ingredients. Thicken or this as needed while cooking. Can serve over rice, if desired.

Powerfully Pregnant

Thai Coconut Soup
(Tracy Slack)

1 Tbsp Olive Oil
2 Tbsp minced Ginger (1/8 tsp ginger powder)
1 Tbsp minced (frozen lemon grass
1 Tbsp Chicken paste (or 4 cups Chicken broth but remove milk later)
1 Tbsp fish sauce
1 can (13.5 ounce) coconut milk
½ lb fresh mushrooms, sliced
1 lb medium shrimp, peeled and de-veined. (Can substitute chicken, fish or mix)
1 Tbsp Lime juice
¼ chopped, fresh cilantro (optional)

Meatballs
(Elizabeth Bailey)

Mix together:
6 lb ground Turkey
Real Salt to taste
A lot of minced, dried Onion
4 Eggs, well beaten
Worcestershire Sauce
Pizza Seasoning
Rolled Oats
Form into balls and bake @ 350' until well done
Or drop into cooking soups.

Nachos
(Rebecca Dimick)

1 lb Hamburger
½ C chopped Onion
¼ chopped Mushrooms
1 tsp Real Salt, Pepper, Garlic powder
1 tsp mild Chili powder (leave out if you have any signs of heat sensitivity)
1 can Black Beans, drained
1 can Kidney Beans, drained
1 C chopped tomatoes
2 Tbs fresh cilantro, chopped
½ C shredded cheese
Instructions:
Preheat oven, to 350'. Brown hamburger with onion, mushrooms, garlic powder, salt, pepper and chili powder. On 9X12 baking sheet layer meat, beans, tomatoes, cilantro and cheese. Bake until cheese is melted. Serve on lightly salted rice cakes or serve as a topping for salad.

Split Pea Soup
(Elizabeth Bailey)

Dry Split Peas
Water
Carrots
Celery
Onions
Bay leaf
Real Salt and Pepper

Southwest Style Bean Dish
(Rebecca Dimick)

1 Can Black Beans
1 Can Kidney Beans
1 Can Whole Corn, drained
½ cup chopped low acid Tomato
1 tsp Vinegar
1 Tbsp Lemon juice
¼ Cup chopped Olives (optional)
2 Tbsp fresh, chopped Cilantro
1 tsp Black Pepper

In medium / large dish combine beans, corn, onion, tomato, olives, cilantro and pepper and stir well until mixed. Pour vinegar and vinegar over ingredients and stir again. May serve warm or cold. Can serve as a side dish or a yummy topping for a salad.

Beef Ribs
(Elizabeth Bailey)

Mix:
Molasses
Real Salt
Vinegar
Chili powder
Black pepper
Old Bay
Thyme
Onion powder
Honey
Garlic

Pour over ribs. Cover with foil and cook at low heat until meat falls off the bone.

Lemon Pepper Baked Salmon
(Rebecca Dimick)

1 Fillet fresh Salmon
1-2 cup Water
2 Tbsp Lemon juice
1 Tbsp Lemon Pepper
1 tsp dried Rosemary
1 tsp Real Salt

Preheat oven to 350'. In 9X12 baking dish place fillet, skin down/ Add water, lemon juice, lemon pepper, Rosemary and salt. Bake 40-60 minutes. Serve with wild rice & steamed vegetables.

Italian Wedding Soup
(Elizabeth Bailey)

1 bag Collards
Garlic
Onion, chopped
Beef Broth
White Beans
Meatballs

        Good eating!!

Powerfully Pregnant

Pecan Crust Rack of Lamb
(Tracy Slack)

½ Cup Dijon Mustard
2 Tbsp Honey
2 Tbsp Molasses
4 Cloves Garlic
1 (3 ½ lb.) Rack of Lamb
2 Cups finely chopped Pecans
1 tsp. chopped Marjoram (1/3 tsp if dried)
¼ Cup Olive Oil
Salt and Pepper to taste (Continued on next page)

Combine mustard, honey, molasses and garlic. Marinate the lamb in this mixture, refrigerated, for at least 4 hours, preferably overnight. Reserve marinade. Next day, bring lamb to room temperature. Allow 4-6 hours. Preheat oven to 400 degrees. Place meat on sheet pan and roast for 8 minutes. Remove and let set for 10 minutes. Meanwhile, combine pecans, marjoram, oil, salt and pepper. Dip Lamb in marinade and dredge in dry ingredients. Bake in bottom of oven until done.

Maple-Pecan Sweet Potatoes
(Tracy Slack)

2½ lbs Sweet Potatoes, peeled and cubed
½ Cup Maple Syrup
3 Tbsp Butter
½ tsp Cinnamon
¼ tsp Cloves
½ Cup Pecans, shopped and toasted

In saucepan, over high heat, bring sweet potatoes and enough salted water to cover to a boil; reduce heat. Once cooked until completely tender, mash with hand potato masher. Mash until smooth. Stir in maple syrup, butter and spices. Sprinkle with toasted pecans.

Onion Rings
(Donna Young)

1 large onion, sliced into rings
6 Tbsp Cream of Wheat
2 tsp Garlic powder
Salt and Pepper to taste
2 eggs
1-2 oz almond or rice milk

Preheat oven to 425'. Cover baking sheet with foil and spray with Olive oil. Milk and eggs thoroughly into one bowl and the dry ingredients into the second bowl. Dip rings into the wet mixture then into the dry mixture, shaking off excess, then lay on the baking sheet. Bake for 15 minutes then turn them over and bake for an additional 5 minutes.

Variation: Add other seasonings into the appropriate bowl (wet or dry) such as Worcestershire sauce, onion salt, dill, mustard, honey etc. Use different veggies such as cauliflower, broccoli, zucchini, any wholesome vegetables. Skewered and grilled is good. Be careful and do not over cook those veggies!

Powerfully Pregnant

~~~~~SALADS~~~~~

Fabulous Fall Salad
(Wendy Ray)

Amounts are approximate: Adjust to your preference and the ingredients you have on hand.
6 Apples, cored and diced into 1.4" chunks
4-6 stalks Celery, sliced into long strips and then cut into ¼" chunks
½ C chopped Walnuts
½ C dried Cranberries or finely diced fresh cranberries.
Optional: Raisins or diced pineapple
2 to 4 Tbsp Blender Mayonnaise or Cashew Cream (Also in this section)
Optional Sweeten with apple or cranberry-apple juice concentrate.

Mom's Waldorf Salad
(Tracy Slack)

Combine:
2 Cups red or green apples, unpeeled & chopped
1 Cup or 2 Ribs Celery, chopped
¼ - ½ Cup Walnuts, broken
¼ Cup Raisins

Dressing:
1 Tbsp Honey
½ tsp lemon juice
¼ Cup Mayo
¼ Cup Fruit Juice
Dash Real Salt

Fruit Rice Salad
(Tracy Slack)

3 Cups cooked short grain brown Rice
2 Cups chunk canned fruit or fresh fruit -- halved grapes, chopped apples, carrots or other fruits (if fresh, soak in ¼ C maple syrup for a while to produce juice. Reserve liquid.
2 Cups sliced Celery
2 Cups Cooked Chicken, cut into bite size pieces.
¾ Cup Blender Mayonnaise
Real Salt to taste.
Combine rice, fruit, celery and chicken. Blend ½ cup reserved fruit juice with blender mayonnaise. Add rice and chicken mixture. Toss lightly. Serves 6.

Chicken Salad
(Elizabeth Bailey)

Mix together:
Roast Chicken leftovers
Homemade cucumber dressing
Prepared Brown Mustard
Chopped Onion
Chopped Apple
Real Salt to taste
Serve with lettuce, rice cakes or corn tortillas.

Powerfully Pregnant

Quinoa Salad with Dried Fruit &Nuts
(Julie Mott)

1 ½ Cups Quinoa
¼ tsp Salt
3 ½ Cups Water
1 bunch Green Onions, chopped
¾ Cup Celery, chopped
½ Cup Raisins
1 pinch Mild Chili Powder (continued on next page)
1 Tbsp mild Olive oil
1 Tbsp Vinegar
2 Tbsp Lemon juice
2 Tbsp Sesame oil
1/3 Cup fresh Cilantro, chopped
¾ Cup Pecans, chopped

Bring the quinoa, salt and water to a boil in a saucepan. Reduce heat to medium-low, cover and simmer until quinoa is tender, 20-25 minutes. Once done, scrape into larger bowl and allow to cool for 20 minutes. Stir in green onions, celery, raisins, chili powder, olive oil, vinegar, lemon juice and sesame oil. Allow to stand at room temperature for 1 hour to allow all flavors to blend. Stir in cilantro and pecans before serving.

Favorite Cole Slaw
(Tracy Slack)

Dressing
½ C Homemade Mayo
¼ C Vinegar
¼ C Agave nectar (or honey or pure maple syrup)
¼ tsp Real Salt
1/8 tsp Black Pepper

4 C or ½ head shredded Cabbage (try ½ purple and ½ green!)
¼ C grated Carrot
2 Tbsp golden raisins
1 small can white chestnuts (optional) 1/8 tsp poppy seeds

Combine dressing ingredients and whisk until smooth. Add cabbage and remaining ingredients and toss well. Refrigerate overnight in a plastic or ceramic container (Do not use metal)

Chicken Salad on Rice Cakes
(Tracy Slack)

2 C cubed Cooked Chicken
1 C diced Cheese
½ C Seedless Grapes cut in half OR
½ C diced Pears
½ C Bender Mayonnaise
¼ C sliced Celery
¼ C raw Sunflower Seeds (unsalted)
¼ tsp Real salt
¼ tsp Pepper

Mix together and place on top of Brown Wild Rice Cakes!

Powerfully Pregnant

Confetti Salad
(Donna Young)

Put into large bowl:
2 Cups cooked Brown / Wild Rice Blend
1 can Black Beans, drained & rinsed
1 bunch Green Onions, sliced
1 Avocado, diced
½ cup frozen Corn
¼ cup Red Bell Pepper, diced
½ cup Cauliflower, cut into small pieces
½ cup broccoli, cut into small pieces

In pint jar, mix:
¾ cup olive oil
¾ cup Apple Cider Vinegar
1 ½ tsp Italian Seasoning (or equal parts thyme and oregano)
½ tsp Real Salt
Shake well and pour over ingredients in bowl. Gently stir together. Serve as a side dish or add 2 cups cooked chicken for a main dish!!

Variety: Use whatever veggies you have on hand that will make it pretty and taste yummy! Exchange kidney beans for black beans. Lots of choices.

Tracy's Carrot Salad
(Tracy Slack)

3 handfuls of shredded carrots
1 Tbsp Pure Maple Syrup
1 Tbsp Lemon Juice
2 Tbsp chopped Pecans
2 Tbsp Raisins
Dash Real Salt

Stir together and serve.

Notes_____
_____
_____
_____
_____
_____
_____
_____
_____
_____
_____

~~~~~DRESSINGS, SPREADS, MISC~~~~~

Almond or Cashew Milk
(Wendy Ray)

1 C Almonds (may be soaked over night to make easier to blend) or Cashews
¼ tsp Salt
2- 4 dates (may be soaked prior to soften)
OR 1-3 Tbsp Honey
Blend in blender until creamy, then pour half of this paste into a small cup. Add 4-5 cups water to the half in the blender. Blend 10 seconds. Pour into pitcher. Repeat with the other half of the paste. Making just over two quarts, total.
May be strained (we actually love the extra fiber and nutty chunks in most things). Serve chilled and stirred.

Carob Milk
(Elizabeth Bailey)

2 ¾ Cup Vanilla Rice Milk or Almond Milk
3 Tbsp Carob powder
Stevia to taste
*optional-- a couple drops of almond extract.
(optional, but very nice!)

Not Egg Nog
(Elizabeth Bailey)

4 egg yolks beaten till light in color and texture
Beat in:
1/3 Cup Honey
3 Cup Rice Milk or Almond Milk
1 tsp. Nutmeg powder
Stir over double boiler till thick.
Chill and serve

Hickory-Honey Mustard
(great mayo alternative)
(Elizabeth Bailey)

3 cups Honey
4 cups cider vinegar
12 Eggs, beaten
1 ½ cups yellow mustard powder
1 tsp Real Salt
1 tsp Garlic
¼ tsp paprika
7 tsp paprika
7 tsp Hickory flavor
3 tsp. mild Chili powder
Cook in a double boiler until thick. Strain and chill

Cashew Cream / Spread
(Wendy Ray)

Place in blender
1 C raw Cashews or almonds
½ to ¾ C Water (just enough to cover nuts)
1-2 Tbsp Honey (liquid state, not crystallized)
1 tsp Real salt

Blend on medium or high speed until creamy. Then with blender still running on medium speed, slowly drizzle 1 cup light olive oil. Do not stop the blender during this process and do not stop it as the oil begins to puddle at the top, so it will not break (into a separated mess--if it does you can still use it to flavor soups, cereals and desserts). Will thicken a bit when refrigerated.

Some uses for this recipe:
- In leftovers from a once warm meal it stays creamy, unlike butter or cream: No cold grease texture.
- So yummy on beans and rice, yams (served warm or cold), on steamed carrots, corn or broccoli!
- Make a ranch dressing: Add ¼ to ½ tsp Garlic powder, ½ to 1 tsp onion powder, ¼ tsp paprika, 1 Tbsp dried parsley (or 3 T fresh parsley) and ¼ tsp dried celery seeds or leaves. Optional: sweeten, add lemon juice.
- Serve over Cranberry Sauce or Baked Apples
- Blend with sliced frozen bananas, berried… sweetening if needed to make "Ice Cream"
- Make creamy soups: Add a few spoonfuls after soup is done
- Add to rice mil to give rich taste

Seasoning Salt-No MSG!
(Elizabeth Bailey)

8 Tbsp Real Salt
3 Tbsp Pepper
2 Tbsp Paprika
½ Tbsp Onion powder
½ Tbsp Garlic Salt

Pizza Seasoning Mix
(Elizabeth Bailey)

Mix these dried herbs:
Onion
Garlic
Oregano
Basil
Parsley
Fennel Seed
Thyme
Marjoram
Celery Seed

BBQ Dry Rub for Meats
(Elizabeth Bailey)

Honey or Molasses
Garlic powder
Paprika
Mild Chili powder
Real Salt

Steak Marinade
(Elizabeth Bailey)

Balsamic Vinegar
Minced Garlic
Black Pepper
Old Bay Seasoning
Real Salt
Pour over meat. Cover. Refrigerate a minimum of 1 hour - -stirring often.
Grill.

Meat Sauce
(Elizabeth Bailey)

2 Cups Honey
1 Cup Molasses
1 Cup Vinegar
½ Tbsp Real Salt
2 Tbsp Garlic
2 Tbsp dried, minced Onion
1 Tbsp Hickory Smoke Flavor
1 Tbsp Turmeric
1 Tbsp Paprika
Simmer to blend flavors.
Refrigerate.
Makes about 1 quart.

Molasses Baked Beans
(Elizabeth Bailey)

Dried Beans, Red, Black and White
(I mix beans for optimum nutrition)
Water
Molasses
Vinegar
Real Salt
Powder Mustard
Chopped Onion

Blender Mayonnaise
(Tracy Slack)

1 Egg
1 scant tsp prepared Mustard
¼ tsp Real salt
1 cup light Olive Oil
3 tsp fresh Lemon juice
 Preparation:
Put the egg, mustard, salt in a blender or food processor; blend at high speed about 20 seconds. Gradually add the oil through the top of the blender, while blending. Drizzle in slowly, blending in all the oil with the egg. Continue to blend until mixture is thick and creamy. Blend in lemon juice last, just until blended. Note: Raw eggs can contain salmonella (about 1 in 20,000 eggs might be contaminated). Those with compromised immune systems may want to use an egg substitute instead of the egg.

Veggie Dip
(Tracy Slack)

To make veggie dip add any, or a combination, of these into the blender mayonnaise.
2 tsp Agave nectar or honey
½ tsp Vinegar
1 tsp Garlic powder (or ½ tsp fresh minced garlic
½ tsp Dill
½ tsp dried Parsley
½ tsp Onion powder
½ tsp Real salt
1 tsp dried Oregano

Variations are endless!!

Pumpkin Butter
(Elizabeth Bailey)

9 cups pumpkin puree
3 cups Honey
1 ½ tsp Cinnamon
¾ tsp. Cloves

Homemade Blender Mayonnaise
(Wendy Ray)

Mix briefly in blender:
3 Eggs
2 Tbsp Lemon juice or raw Apple Cider Vinegar
Then add:
1 tsp Real salt
1 Tbsp Honey (or substitute) Optional
½ tsp Mustard powder

Blend in blender or food processor on medium speed until honey is dissolved. With blender still running, slowly pour in about one cup light olive oil. (amount will vary depending on amount of water used to puree the nuts)
You are done when it starts to puddle on top of the mayonnaise. If over blended the cream may break. It will continue to thicken as it cools. Keep refrigerated.

Honey Mustard Dressing
(Wendy Ray)

½ cup Honey
1/3 cup Raw Apple Cider Vinegar
1 teaspoon Real Salt
1 to 2 Tbsp prepared Mustard
1 slice Onion (purple makes it pretty!)
Or 2 tsp Onion Powder

Whip in a blender, then drizzle one cup Olive oil (virgin olive oil is usually too strong for this recipe) with the blender still going. Then stir in parsley flakes and paprika (or poppy seeds, Italian seasonings, get creative!!)

Zucchini Pickles
(Elizabeth Bailey)

14-16 small zucchini, sliced (mix yellow and green)
8 small onions, slices
2 medium green bell peppers, sliced
Sprinkle 1/3 C Real salt into the veggies in a bowl and mix well. Top it off with ice cubes and let it set out for 1 ½ hours.
Then rinse well and drain.

Mix in large pan:
2 C Honey
2 Tbsp Mustard seed
1 Tbsp dry Mustard
1 tsp Turmeric
1 tsp Celery seed
1 tsp Peppercorns
3 C Cider Vinegar

Bring to boil and add veggies and boil again. Simmer 10 minutes. Pack quart jars to neck. Clean tops, put on clean warm lids. Water bath 25 minutes.

Sweet Pickled Beets
(Donna Young)

Leaving about 2 inches of tops on the roots, cook beets until skins slip easily. Put into cold water them remove skins and tops from roots. Cut, if they are too big, into smaller pieces 1-1 ½ inch pieces. Pack beets into jars up to the neck.

Syrup:
Mix well and bring to a boil…
2 C Honey
3 C Water
3 C Apple Cider Vinegar
1 tsp Clove, powder
1 tsp Allspice, powder
1 Tbsp Cinnamon, powder

Pour boiling syrup over beets to cover beets. Clean top of jars and put new lids on then fasten on with rings. Water bath for 30 minutes for quarts. They will be ready to eat in about two weeks.

Fruit Syrup for Canning
(Donna Young)

When canning fruit a healthy heavy syrup can be made by using 5 parts water and 1 part honey. Stir together and heat on stovetop until honey and water are mixed thoroughly and mixture comes to just under a boil. (If allowed to boil, it will cause a foam) Use this syrup instead of sugar to can fruits with.

Strawberry Jam
(Donna Young)

Wash strawberries, remove tops and mash with potato masher. Sweeten with honey or agave nectar to taste. Measure strawberries, into large heavy pan, and for every 4 cups of berry mix, add 1 tsp of Fruit Fresh and 1 box of Sure-Gel in the pink box (this one does not require sugar for thickening). Put on heat and bring to a boil. Let boil for 3 minutes then put directly into clean, pint jars. Clean tops of jars and put on warm, new lids. Jars should seal in 30 minutes or so if the jam was very hot when lid was put on. Lots of other jams can be made using the same process. We have made peach, apricot and pear. Use a little more fruit or less Sure-Gel to make it a little thinner for syrup.

Gingerbread
(Elizabeth Bailey)

Mix and bake:
5 Cups Rolled oats
3 cups Water
1 tsp Real Salt
3 Tbsp Baking powder
¼ cup Olive oil
½ cup Agave
3 Eggs
1 cup Molasses
1 tsp cloves
1 tsp Cinnamon
1 tsp Ginger

Batter Bread
(Elizabeth Bailey)

Stir together:
5 Cups Raw Rolled Oats
3 Cups Water or Rice Milk
1 tsp. Real Salt
3 Tbsp Baking Powder
¼ cup Honey
¼ cup Olive Oil
3 Eggs
Put in oiled loaf pan.
Bake @ 350' till golden and set.
This is gluten free and very crumbly. Cut thick makes a passable open faced sandwich.

Cinnamon Raisin Bread
(Elizabeth Bailey)

Same as recipe above, then add:
1 Cup Raisins
1 Tbsp Cinnamon
Drizzle with Honey before baking.

Cornbread
(Elizabeth Bailey)

2 Cups Cornmeal
4 Tbsp Honey
4 tsp Baking Powder
1 tsp Real Salt
1 cup Rice Milk
1 Egg
¼ cup Olive Oil
Pour into oiled pan, bake @ 350' till golden brown. Crumbly, but tastes good. Especially if you go a little heavy on the honey.

Powerfully Pregnant

~~~~~DESSSERTS AND TREATS~~~~~

Brownies
(Dean & Mande Land)

These are the best brownies we have ever tasted! Note: Do not exchange honey for the agave, it does not give the right texture.

16 oz jar Creamy Almond Butter
2 Eggs
1 ¼ C Agave Nectar
1 Tbsp Vanilla Extract
½ Cacao Powder
1 Cup chopped walnuts (or other nuts)
½ tsp Real Salt
1 tsp Baking Powder

Mix together and bake at 350 degrees for 35 to 40 minutes.

Peanut Butter Cookies
(Elizabeth Bailey)

1 ½ Cup Peanut Butter
¾ Cup Honey
3 Tbsp Lecithin Powder
1 Cup Raw Rolled Oats

Roll into teaspoon sized balls
Flatten with fork or make thumbprints and fill with homemade jam. Also can be sprinkled with cinnamon.

Macaroons
(Elizabeth Bailey)

3 Cups shredded, unsweetened coconut
½ tsp. Real Salt
2 tsp Vanilla extract
2 Egg whites, beaten
2/3 Cup Honey

Drop onto oiled cookie sheet. Bake @ 350' for 20 minutes
Variations:
Drizzle with carob sauce
Stir in almond pieces

Pumpkin Pie
(Elizabeth Bailey)

1 large can Pumpkin puree
1 tsp Real Salt
1 cup Honey
1 tsp Pumpkin pie spices
6 eggs, beaten.

Mix together until smooth. Pour into one of the Almond or Oatmeal pie shells in this section and bake at 350F until set.

Cranberry Sauce
(Donna Young)

1 bag (12 oz.) Fresh Cranberries
1 cup Honey

Wash cranberries and sort. In pan, put cranberries and honey. Bring to a boil and continue to boil until berries 'pop' and then the mixture thickens. Remove from heat. It can be used fresh and warm or it is wonderful cold and canned. To bottle: Remove from heat and immediately pour into clean pint jar. Clean top of jar with clean, damp cloth and put on new warm lid with ring. It should seal within a few minutes.

Cranberry-Apple Dessert
Dad's favorite 'Cherry' Dessert
(Donna Young)

1 pint cranberry sauce (*recipe above*)
4 apples, peeled and diced or sliced
½ cup Honey
4 Tbsp Cornstarch
1 cup Water
1 tsp Vanilla extract
½ tsp Cinnamon
Optional: ½ cup Raisins or Currants

Pour cranberry sauce, honey and apples into large pan. Mix cornstarch into water and when completely dissolved, pour into pan with fruit and honey. Bring to a boil, stirring constantly and cook till mixture thickens. Add Vanilla and Cinnamon.
Topping
 Mix 1 cup old fashioned rolled oats, ½ cup chopped nuts and stir in enough honey to make oat mixture 'sticky', then sprinkle with ½ tsp cinnamon. Place in a thin layer in a pan and put in the oven on Low Broil, stirring frequently, until mix becomes slightly dry and crunchy. Remove from heat. Serve warm or cold topped with oat topping.

Strawberry Ice Cream
(Melissa Morgan)

1- 10 oz pkg Frozen Strawberries
1- 13.5 oz can Coconut milk
¼ cup Agave Nectar
1 Tbsp Vanilla extract
½ tsp Vanilla Bean (optional)
½ tsp Coconut extract

Blend all ingredients in blender. Pour into ice cream maker and process according to directions.

Peach Nutty Ice Cream
(Tracy Slack)

1 C raw Cashews (or almonds, walnuts, pecans etc)
3 C diced fresh (or canned without sugar or corn syrup) Peaches
½ C Pure Maple Syrup, Agave Nectar or Honey
1 tsp vanilla extract
 Place nuts in food processor or blender and grind to powder (do not over grind or you get nut butter) Add remaining ingredients and blend until peaches are the consistency you want. Freeze in ice cream maker according to manufacturer's directions. Enjoy!! Will be very hard if you just put it in the freezer. Recipe can be modified with any type of fruit... .strawberries, apricots, etc.

Caramel Apples
(Holt Young)

6 Medium, fresh Apples
2 cups Honey
1 cup Peanut Butter
1 tsp. Vanilla extract
½ cup chopped Nuts, if desired

Wash the apples, dry them well and put craft sticks into the end of the apples for handles then set the apples aside until later.

Put 2 cups honey in a heavy pan. Bring to a boil and let boil until it comes to a soft ball stage. Be careful not to over cook the honey. My mom taught me how to do a water test on the honey. It is where you take some cold water in a cup and when you think he honey is about right you put a little spoonful in the water and it will cool and show you what it will be like when it is finished. Then if you want to cook it more you can or you can stop when it is right. When the honey is at a soft ball stage then remove it from the heat and add 1 cup of peanut butter and stir until it is mixed well. Be careful not to get burned. After the peanut butter is mixed in then add a teaspoon of vanilla and stir again. Once everything is stirred together then hold the apples by their handles and, one at a time, dip them into the honey and peanut butter caramel. Use a spoon to drip the caramel over the tops but not on the handles. Then dip them into chopped nuts, if you want to.

We also like the apples sliced with the caramel drizzled over the top, sprinkled with either nuts or shredded coconut!! Here's a secret: This same caramel can be used to make popcorn balls!! ☺

Cool Treats
(Wendy Ray)

In our neighborhood it's not uncommon for all the wandering kids to have 6 sugared pops (or something like that) every day. They get one from their parents, one from the grandma down the street, one from each friend's house.... I don't know about everyone else, but that is NOT okay! Our children, by the way, do little wandering, and we are fortunate to live on the edge of the wilderness, so it's not too hard to keep them close, but sometimes a friend will bring an armful to share. >:(

SO... We've been fighting back. Our ammunition?

Frozen grapes!!!! They are not very messy, they don't stick together in the freezer bag, they're easy to divide and share, they're cold. Best of all, they're food!

Other favorites:
Frozen 100% juice in popsicle molds with plastic spoons for sticks! (okay, juice is still sugar, but it's better)
Ice cubes (surprisingly, the most popular!)
Frozen bananas on a stick (sometimes rolled in nuts before freezing)
Frozen leftover green smoothies (which are usually more of a purple or an almost-chocolaty brown, really, depending on the fruits we put in)
Frozen almond milk (usually with bananas and flax blended in)

If I'm too busy to supervise any of that, there's always the parsley, spinach or kale that they're constantly mowing down - almost all the kids in the neighborhood like them!
Here's to a cool summer

Mixed Berry Crisp
(Tracy Slack)

6 Cups mixed Berries (your choice of blackberries, raspberries, blueberries, strawberries etc)
6 Tbsp Tapioca
2 Tbsp Pure Maple Syrup

Preheat oven to 350 degrees. Wash fruit and drain well. Cut off tops of strawberries and halve. If using frozen fruit leave whole, thaw until separated an drain off excess juices well. Transfer to large mixing bowl. Fold in tapioca and drizzle with maple syrup. Mix well. Pour into oiled baking dish.

Topping
2 Cups Rolled Oats
½ Cup Wheat Germ or Wheat Bran
¼ tsp Real Salt
½ tsp Cinnamon
½ Cup Light Olive Oil
3 Tbsp liquid Maple Syrup

Combine oats, wheat germ, salt and cinnamon in mixing bowl. Combine oil and maple syrup in measuring cup and add to oat mixture. Mix well. Sprinkle topping over berry mix evenly. Bake uncovered 30 minutes at 350 degrees or until fruit juices bubble up around edges or through the cracks. Remove from heat and cool until it sets. Serve with whipped coconut cream.

Granola Style Popcorn balls
(Wendy Ray)

We have a favorite family treat that is pretty healthy, but it hit me yesterday that I could use coconut oil in place of the butter! It was fantastic! Not greasy or sticky, but still formed into crispy, minimally messy balls. Cool. With a fruit smoothie or some cold almond milk on the side, you're set for a healthy party everyone will enjoy... unless they're allergic to nuts, I guess. (in which case you could leave them out and it would still be delicious!)

Popcorn balls, granola style
8 to 12 cups air-popped popcorn (scoop into a large bowl -- with extra room for mixing-- after popping to leave un-popped kernels behind)

Make the syrup:
Bring to a boil (or just enough to melt it if you don't mind it a bit stickier... doesn't make much difference) in a small pan on the stove:

3 Tablespoons coconut oil (It's great for this recipe because it's solid at room temperature, like butter is. I make sure to use cold-pressed from a good source)
¼ cup honey (you could use agave or pure maple syrup, I think)
½ tsp vanilla (and/or 1/8 tsp maple or almond flavoring)
1 teaspoon cinnamon
Pour mixture over popcorn and stir to coat. Add your choice of extras:
1 to 2 cups dried fruits (raisins, apricots, pineapple, currants, dates, etc)
1 to 2 Cups chopped (or not) nuts (peanuts, almonds, cashews, walnuts... Sunflower seeds, pumpkin seeds, coconut, ground flax, etc.)

For a Christmas treat we make one regular batch and another without the cinnamon, but with two drops peppermint oil added to the syrup.

Powerfully Pregnant

Carob Cake
(Skyler Bailey)

2 cups Rolled oats
1 cup Carob powder
1 cup Butter, room temp
2 tsp. Vanilla extract
½ cup honey
2 tsp baking powder
1 cup Rice milk
2 Eggs

Mix well. Pour into olive oiled baking dish and bake at 350F for 35 minutes.

Whipped Coconut Cream
(Donna Young)

This is to replace whipped cream for desserts and such. Coconut cream takes a little longer to whip and it needs to be cold to start with. Put the cream, beaters and glass bowl in the fridge for several hours (or over night) before doing this one. Put your cold coconut cream into a glass bowl and put your mixer on the high speed. Whip until the cream forms soft peaks like whipped cream. Add sweetener to taste and a little vanilla. Note: Lots of varieties on this one, play with your favorites.

Nut & Seed Honey Nut Butter Balls
(Tracy Slack)

4 C ground Nuts, seeds into a butter (or use store bought Nut Butter
1 C dried unsweetened Coconut
2/3 C unsweetened Carob powder
1 ½ C Honey

Mix all ingredients together by hand or in a food processor. Roll into balls. For variety roll in ground nuts, sesame seeds or coconut. For a crunchy feel add ¼ C nut pieces at end. Refrigerate or freeze. Serve cold.

Popcorn Trail Mix
(Tabitha Newman)

¾ Cup Honey
2 T. Raw, Coconut Oil
½ tsp. Pure Vanilla Extract
1/8 tsp. Real Salt or Sea Salt
½ C. Pop Corn kernels, popped or 10 C. Popped Popcorn
1 C. Almonds, whole
1 C. Dried Cherries (unsweetened)
½ C. Sunflower Seeds
½ C. Pepita's (raw, shelled, pumpkin seeds)
¼ C. Coconut, shredded & unsweetened

Bring honey too a low boil over medium high heat (about 4-5 minutes) until it reaches a soft ball stage. Remove from heat and stir in coconut oil, vanilla, and salt. Let cool to room temperature. In a large bowl combine popped popcorn, almonds, dried cherries, sunflower seeds, pepita's, and coconut. Pour honey mixture over top of mixture and stir until everything is evenly coated. Place in refrigerator for about 30 minutes or until set.
Our family likes to take this trail mix up hiking. It makes for a very nutritious and energizing snack.

Chocolate Oatmeal Haystack Cookie
(Tracy Slack)

2 Cups Maple or Honey granules
½ Cup Coconut Milk
½ Cup Butter
½ Cup Raw Cacao
1/16 tsp Real Salt
½ tsp Vanilla extract
3 Cups Rolled Oats
1 Cup Flaked, chipped or shredded coconut.

Squash seeds
(Elizabeth Bailey)

Remove seeds from squash. Wash and towel dry seeds. Place in one layer on an olive oiled cookie sheet. Sprinkle with Worcestershire Sauce and Real Salt. Toast at 350' till just golden and dry. May stir while baking, careful not to over-roast

Nut Balls
(Tracy Slack)

¾ C Almond Butter
½ Carob powder (optional)
½ tsp Cinnamon
1/3 to ½ C Honey or other natural sweetener
1 tsp Vanilla
1 C puffed Cereal* tiny puffed grain like quinoa or millet
½ C chopped Nuts* any seeds or chopped nuts, like lightly toasted or raw pecan pieces.
Coating options
Unsweetened coconut
Carob powder

Thoroughly combine the almond butter, carob, cinnamon, honey and vanilla. The dough will be quite stiff. Knead in the nuts and cereal. With wet hands, form into walnuts-sized balls. Make sure the surface is glistening damp. Choose which coating you'd like to use and roll balls in either coconut, carob ganache or carob powder. Coconut coating is the nicest and easy to coat by shaking the balls in a ziploc bag with the coconut.
Refrigerate until firm or freeze in an air-tight container to store for a week or more.

Chocolate Peanut Butter Haystacks
(Tracy Slack)

10 oz Agave Chocolate Syrup
10 oz Unsweetened Peanut Butter
10 oz Chipped or shredded Coconut
10 oz Rolled Oats
¾ C Organic Peanuts (or other nut pieces)

No Bake Oatmeal Cookies
(Donna Young)

2 C Honey
1 C Peanut Butter, crunchy
3 C Rolled Oats
½ tsp Real Salt
1 tsp Vanilla Extract

Put honey into a pan and boil to a soft ball stage. Remove from heat and add peanut butter. Stir until mixed. Put rolled oats, vanilla and salt into a bowl. Pour peanut butter and honey mix over oats and stir until thoroughly mixed. Dough should hold shape into a ball….add more oats if needed. Drop by spoonfuls onto wax paper and let cool.

Two layer Peanut Butter and Cacao Pudding
(Donna Young)

Peanut Butter layer:
3 C Almond milk
¼ C Honey or Agave Nectar
¼ C + 1 Tbsp Corn Starch
1 heaping tsp Gelatin
4 Egg yokes, slightly beaten
1/3 C Peanut Butter
1 tsp Vanilla extract.

Mix almond milk, honey, corn starch, gelatin and egg yokes in saucepan. Mix with whisk until thoroughly mixed. Bring to a boil and boil till mixture begins to thicken. Add in peanut butter and vanilla. Stir well then pour into 9x9x2" pan. Set in fridge.

Cacao Layer:
3 C Almond milk
1/3 C honey or agave nectar
¼ C + 1 Tbsp Corn starch
1 heaping tsp Gelatin
4 Egg yokes, slightly beaten
¼ C Cacao powder (or carob)
1 tsp Vanilla extract
1 dropper Chocolate Stevia

Mix almond milk, honey, cornstarch, gelatin, cacao and egg yokes in a saucepan. Mix with whisk until thoroughly mixed and smooth. Bring to a boil and cook until mixture begins to thicken. Add in vanilla and stevia and stir well. Pour on top of peanut butter layer to fill pan. Chill for at least two hours. Serve chilled.

Variations: This recipe can be adjusted to fit coconut cream, banana cream or any other cream pie desired...Play with it and see what you can find.

Can use Tracy's No Bake Almond Pie Shells to make a pie on special occasions.

Fruit Juice Jigglers
(Tracy Slack)

2- 12oz cans 100% Fruit juice
7- 8 Tbsp Plain Beef Gelatin
2 ½ cups COLD Water

In saucepan, being juice just to a boil. Sprinkle Gelatin over water over cold water. Let soak into water a few minutes. Use a whisk if necessary. Pour into saucepan

Fruit Juice Block
(Rachel Brighton)

4 envelopes of unflavored Gelatin
1 cup cold Fruit Juice
3 cups Fruit Juice, heated to boiling
2 Tbsp Honey, optional

1. Sprinkle gelatin over cold juice in large bowl; let stand 1 minute. Add hot juice and stir until gelatin completely dissolves, about 5 minutes. Stir in honey, if desired. Pour into 9X12X2 inch pan
2. Refrigerate until firm, about 3 hours. To serve, cut into 1 inch squares, it's a finger food!

Cranberry Pear Dessert
(Elizabeth Bailey)

In baking dish:
Mix enough Granola, honey, butter and salt together to put a 1 inch layer in baking dish.

Top with a mix of:
1 qt. canned Pears (without sugar)
1- 2 cups whole Cranberries
¼ cup Honey
3 Tbsp Cornstarch
½ tsp Nutmeg
2 Tbsp Molasses

Stir together and pour on top of granola mix. Bake at 350F until bubbly.

Vanilla Bean Ice Cream
(Melissa Morgan)

1 - 10 oz pkg Frozen Strawberries
1- 13.5 oz can Coconut milk
¼ cup Agave Nectar
1 Tbsp Vanilla extract
½ tsp Vanilla Bean (optional)

Blend all ingredients in blender. Pour into ice cream maker and process according to directions.

Hot Real Cacao
(Tracy Slack)

2 Cups Rice or Almond Milk
1 Tbsp 100% Cacao (unsweetened, unprocessed)
¼ Cup Agave Nectar (or honey) approx.
6 drops Chocolate Stevia
1 tsp Vanilla Extract
¼ Cup Coconut Milk (optional)

Put rice / almond milk into a saucepan. Bring almost to a boil. Add cacao powder and whisk until smooth. Turn off heat and add agave, stevia and vanilla. Stir and enjoy! Note: Raw, unprocessed non-alkali cacao is high in antioxidants!

Baked Apples
(Donna Young)

5 large Fuji Apples, peeled and cored
¾ cup of Raisins
½ cup chopped Nuts.
½ tsp Cinnamon
½ tsp Nutmeg
¾ cup of Pure Maple Syrup

Slice apples into a baking dish, mix in raisins and nuts. Sprinkle with cinnamon and nutmeg and drizzle the pure maple syrup over the top. Cover with lid or foil and put in the oven for 35 minutes, or until tender, at 350F.

Toffee Nuts
(Wendy Ray)

Saute until medium brown and bubbly:
1 Tbsp Butter
1 Tbsp Honey
1 Cup Pecans, Walnuts, Cashews, Peanuts or Almonds (chopped or whole)

Stir mixture over medium heat while butter and honey "toffee-ize" (about 3 minutes). A light blue smoke indicates the toffee is done (or in my pans, when it starts to smoke and stick to the bottom of the pan and I'm afraid it'll burn….that's when I know it is perfect). Pour onto glass dish or waxed paper and cool in freezer. Remove whenever you want to use them Great for topping on thick frozen banana-and-almond shakes, apple crisp, salads, popcorn (drizzled with a little melted butter and honey), etc.

Honey Walnut Treats!
(Tracy Slack)

3 Cups Walnuts
3 Tbsp Pure Maple Syrup, or enough to coat.
¼ tsp Real Salt
¼ tsp Cinnamon
Dash Nutmeg (optional)
Dash Allspice (optional)

Mix. Spread evenly on a non-stick baking sheet. Bake @ 350 degrees until it starts to brown. Do NOT overcook. Watch closely so it does not burn. Turn once during baking.

Oatmeal Pie Crust
(Melissa Morgan)

3 C Rolled Oats
½ C sliced Almonds, or other nuts of choice
¼ cup Wheat Germ
2/3 C honey
¼ C light Olive oil
2 Tbsp warm Water
½ tsp Real Salt
1 tsp Vanilla

Preheat oven to 250'. Lightly oil baking sheet. In bowl combine honey, oil, water, salt and vanilla. Stir well; then pour into oat mixture and stir. Spread out on cookie sheet. Bake for 1 hour, stirring every 15 minutes. I also add cinnamon before I bake it and raisins afterward. Good with rice milk.

Almond and Oat Crust
(Tracy Slack)

1 C Almond meal (grind in food processor until fine but not 'butter')
1 C Rolled Oats
3 Tbsp Butter
2 tsp Stevia powder (1/8 tsp if using the 100%)
Drizzle with Pure Maple Syrup or Honey to taste (about 2-3 Tbsp)

Mix and pat into spring form pan (any pan will work but this pan is easier to get product out to serve without falling apart)
I read that this recipe can be cooked but I never cook it. Also some of the crust can be save to crumble on top of the filling!!

No Bake Almond Pie Shells
Similar to a Graham Cracker Crust
(Tracy Slack)

Grind in blender until finely ground:
2 C Almonds
1 C soft Dates (pitted and soaked till soft)
Add:
½ tsp Real salt
½ tsp Vanilla extract

Spray 2 (9") pie plates with non-stick spray. Divide mixture in half and press firmly into plates. Fill with pie filling.

Oat Crust
(Elizabeth Bailey)

Mix together:
1 1/3 Cup Rolled Oats
½ tsp Real Salt
¼ Cup Butter

Sprinkle with cold water, up to 4 Tbsp until it can be formed into a sticky ball. Press into pie plate, fill and bake.

Crock Pot Stewed Apples
(Tracy Slack)

3 lbs Apples, sliced, cored and peeled (or not)
1 tsp Cinnamon
1 dash Nutmeg
3 Tbsp Tapioca
¾ Cup Maple Syrup, honey or granules of either
2 Tbsp Butter

Put first 5 ingredients into crock pot. Stir well to coat apples with the spices. Dot with butter. Cook on low for 4 to 6 hours. Stir once during cooking. Since crock pot temperatures vary, you should check to make sure that apples are soft but not mushy. It should have the consistency of apple pie filling.

Banana Colada Ice Cream
(Holt Young)

3 cups frozen, sliced Bananas
2/3 cup Coconut milk
1/3 cup shredded Coconut, unsweetened
8 drops Orange Stevia
8 drops Vanilla Crème Stevia

Blend until smooth. Serve immediately

~~~~~KNOW YOUR INGREDIENTS~~~~~

Agave Nectar is an acceptable, natural sweetener. The texture is similar to a thin honey but it has a more mild flavor. Most recipes will exchange with honey by equal parts. Agave can be sweeter.

Beef gelatin is a high protein food that is easily assimilated in the body. It is a good choice for those who have difficulties digesting meats. Gelatin can be used in many desserts as well as soups, stews as well as other entrees. Gelatin can be used to thicken many cold dishes as it melts just above 100 degrees and thickens upon cooling.

Butter should be used in small amounts to avoid the raising of cholesterol in the body and avoiding liver issues. However, butter is preferred over margarines. Just do not over do.

Cacao is a raw, unprocessed chocolate powder that does not harm the liver the way most chocolate does. It is generally more preferred for flavor than carob and is still healthy.

Canned Fruit would mean canned without sugar or artificial sweeteners.

Carob is a evergreen tree that tastes similar to chocolate. It is not as smooth flavored as cocoa or cacao but is the healthiest of the three. Sold in a powder and used as a baking cocoa replacement.

Cheeses fall into different categories. As they are a dairy product they carry some of the problems noted in animal milk. Soft cheese such as Cream or Cottage Cheese carry many of the same problems as cow's milk. Harder, block cheeses tend to have enough positive benefits to warrant their use as often as 4-5 times per week. Block (Hard) cheeses do not tend to cause morning sickness or infections like the other dairy products therefore become acceptable fairly frequently.

Coconut cream is made by pressing the flesh of a freshly opened coconut. It is a thick cream that is comparable to whipping cream. It can be gotten, in small amounts, by letting the coconut milk set in a wide mouth container in the refrigerator until it is cold. Once the cream separates it will rise to the top and can be skimmed off. Use the remaining for recipes that do not require the high fat content of the cream.

Curry Powder, like all heat producing spices, should be used very sparingly during the summer months and with anyone who has excess heat in the body. Signs of excess heat could be hot flashes, fevers, red complexion, headaches, irritations of the eyes, ears, nose or throat, bruising or bleeding with brushing teeth or nosebleeds as well as frustration, irritability or anger. Omit curry powder if any of these symptoms exist.

Flour is a ground grain. Grains were intended to do their work in the digestive tract for the purpose of fiber and some nutrients not intended to cross the intestinal/blood barrier. Once the grain has been ground to a flour state the particles then cross that barrier and store in the body as fat as well as damage certain organs and glands. It is preferred to use grains in a whole, cracked, or rolled state. Ground nut flour (almond, coconut, etc) are more acceptable but still need to be consumed no more than 2-3 times per week. Fresh state is better than the dried 'flour' state.

Garlic is a therapeutic spice and is not considered a heat producer. High in antioxidants as well as being anti-viral, anti-parasitic, anti-bacterial and anti-fungal. Very healthy for the immune system. Use freely

Lemon Juice is high acid and should be used in small quantities unless the body ph is tested to be in the alkaline levels. The amounts in these recipes are acceptable for one of two reasons. 1) Those who are testing for high alkaline levels and need the extra acid intake to balance their ph levels or 2) The recipes have the lemon juice diluted. Water has a ph of 7, which is neutral, and the dilution brings the acid level down to a friendly level for human consumption.

Maple Syrup is pure maple syrup and is an acceptable sweetener.

Meats are a good source of protein. Beef, all poultry, all fish, lamb, most wild game are acceptable. The only meats we object to are pork, processed meats (like bologna etc) and meats that are raised with hormones and antibiotics. Clean meat is always preferred over those that have had chemicals, vaccinations and toxins. If the source of the meat is not known to be without the aforementioned then the meat should always be cooked completely to avoid health problems.

Milk, in a recipe, refers to Rice, Almond or Coconut milk. Animal milk is not used during pregnancy.

Molasses is a natural sweetener that has a strong flavor to it. Generally is not used as a replacement for honey or agave due to the strong flavor. It is usually used in smaller amounts to compliment the other sweeteners however it is acceptable and can be used freely.

Nuts are best raw and shelled unless otherwise stated to maintain the nutritional values.

Olive Oil is made in different grades. The darker it is the stronger the flavor. The light colored is generally very mild in flavor and goes in recipes where the stronger flavor is not needed. Personal choice is the best decision maker for the one you want. Most recipes call for the milder flavor.

Onions are used for flavor and have a lot of therapeutic value to them. They are not considered a heat producer and are encouraged often. Loaded with vitamins and antioxidants.

Peppers are used for flavoring other foods, as a rule. Sweet peppers can be eaten as often as desired in everything from stews, soups to casseroles, salads and meat dishes. There are no limits to how many sweet peppers a person should eat. Very high in vitamins and antioxidants.

Heat producing peppers (cayenne, chili, jalapeno, habanera etc) are not acceptable as they produce a reaction in the body that increases the chances of inflammations and bleeding. (*See more on this in the diet section*)

Potatoes should be used only sparingly because the starch stores in the body and causes a lot of weight gain on mother and child. Potatoes should not be eaten more than 1-2 times per week. Sweet potatoes can be substituted in most recipes and are acceptable without limits.

Rolled Oats refers to Old Fashioned rolled oats unless otherwise stated.

Salt means Real Salt, or mined rock salt that has not been heated or processed, just ground down. Mined salt is generally more free of modern day contaminants than sea salt and has more of the stabilized minerals than table salt.

Stevia is a plant with a very sweet leaf. The leaf is green and is sometimes sold as a green powder. This leaf is sweet but it does not break down well in liquids. It also has a difficult time penetrating other dry ingredients for even distribution. Stevia is also sold in a white powder that breaks down immediately in liquids. It also is available in a liquid that can be gotten in plain or different flavored that is used by the drops. Stevia is acceptable.

Sweet potatoes / Yams are in the vegetable category and can be eaten as often as desired. Both can be used in recipes that call for potatoes and enjoyed the same. Mashed, baked, in stews and desserts they are an extremely versatile and healthy food.

Vanilla means the extract of the vanilla bean, not artificial flavoring.

Vinegar unless stated otherwise, means apple cider vinegar, due to the therapeutic value in it. Vinegar is diluted to 5.5-6.5 pH which is friendly.

NOTES

Powerfully Pregnant

~~~~~A Short Story~~~~~

I was objecting to the price of groceries to one of my adult sons. He stood quietly as I told him. It cost so much and there was nothing to show for it. There was no car, no house, no horse, nothing! "It is such a waste of money".

He looked at me with a smile and said "Mom, you have the healthiest family I have ever known. There is less illness in your household than anywhere. This has to be the best health insurance money can buy and it is more effective than any other policy out there and it tastes good. Who else can say that about their health insurance?"

I realized he was right. We do eat well and it is not as expensive as being sick or having sickness within the home. It had been so long since we had a sick person in our house that I forgot and begun to take our health for granted. This was wrong of me and I was humbled to be put back on track by my son who was paying more attention.

~~~~A Short Story~~~~~

When arriving at a birth, early one morning, we found that our laboring mother was extremely pale. She was a blue eyed blond that had no pink in her cheeks or across her nose and her skin was bleached out. This was a surprise as she had never shown problems like this before. I took her blood pressure and it was 90/40, which is too low to go into labor as the body is prone to bleed excessively with too low blood pressure. I asked her if she had started bleeding yet and she told me she had passed a little blood just minutes before.

I had her take four tablespoons of a good liquid calcium every 10 - 15 minutes for about an hour and by then the contractions had quit. During that time her husband mixed up a quart of electrolytes and she drank that, then fell asleep.

When the grocery store opened, (yes, small town) he went and got two bags of spinach. He brought them home and blended one of them up with fruit juice and she drank it. She rested a while and then got up to have lunch. By this time the blood pressure was up to 100/ 48 and she was still pale and was still spotting.

Mid afternoon her husband blended the other bag of spinach with fruit juice for her and she drank it. There had been no contractions since early morning which gave her time to work on the issues at hand. She now had the bleeding completely stopped.

Early evening her blood pressure was at 110/60 but she was feeling tired, in spite of the naps she had. She was given a little oxygen support and she responded right away. Within 10 minutes she went into labor. After a five hour labor, she gave birth to a beautiful baby boy. She had plenty of strength for labor, no excess bleeding and looked beautiful as she latched her new son on for his first meal.

Notes_____

_____

_____

_____

_____

Made in the USA
Middletown, DE
10 May 2024